0982306

BRITISH MEDICAL ASSOCIATION

WITHDRAWN
FROM LIBRARY

KT-427-755

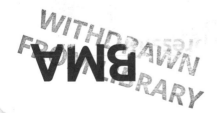

WITHDRAWN
FROM LIBRARY
BMA

WILEY Blackwell

BMJ|Books

www.abcbookseries.com

official guidelines, please visit:
For more information on all books in the ABC series, including links to further information, references and links to the latest

▶ Full colour photographs and illustrations aid diagnosis and patient understanding of a condition
▶ An easy-to-use resource, covering the symptoms, investigations, treatment and management of conditions presenting in day-to-day practice and patient support
▶ Highly illustrated, informative and a practical source of knowledge

in training and all those in primary care
The ABC series contains a wealth of indispensable resources for GPs, GP registrars, junior doctors, doctors

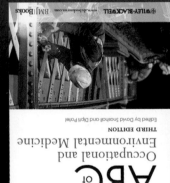

ABC
of
Occupational and
Environmental Medicine
THIRD EDITION
Edited by David Snashall and Dipti Patel

ABC
of
Ear, Nose and Throat
SIXTH EDITION
Edited by Harold Ludman and Patrick J Bradley

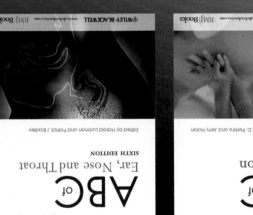

ABC
of
Resuscitation
SIXTH EDITION
Edited by Jasmeet Soar, Gavin D. Perkins and Jerry Nolan

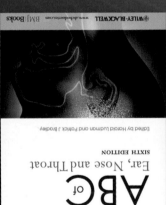

ABC
of
Pain
Edited by Lesley Colvin and Marie Fallon

An outstanding collection of resources for everyone
in primary care

ABC
series

# ABC of

# Anxiety and Depression

EDITED BY

## *Linda Gask*
University of Manchester
Manchester, UK

## *Carolyn Chew-Graham*
Research Institute, Primary Care and Health Sciences and
National School for Primary Care Research, Keele University, Keele, UK

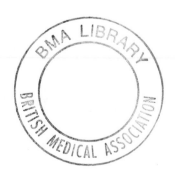

BMA LIBRARY
BRITISH MEDICAL ASSOCIATION

**WILEY** Blackwell

BMJ|Books

This edition first published 2014, © 2014 by John Wiley & Sons, Ltd

BMJ Books is an imprint of BMJ Publishing Group Limited, used under licence by John Wiley & Sons.

*Registered Office:* John Wiley & Sons, Ltd, The Atrium, Southern Gate, Chichester, West Sussex, PO19 8SQ, UK

*Editorial Offices:* 9600 Garsington Road, Oxford, OX4 2DQ, UK
111 River Street, Hoboken, NJ 07030-5774, USA

For details of our global editorial offices, for customer services and for information about how to apply for permission to reuse the copyright material in this book please see our website at www.wiley.com/wiley-blackwell

The right of the author to be identified as the author of this work has been asserted in accordance with the UK Copyright, Designs and Patents Act 1988.

All rights reserved. No part of this publication may be reproduced, stored in a retrieval system, or transmitted, in any form or by any means, electronic, mechanical, photocopying, recording or otherwise, except as permitted by the UK Copyright, Designs and Patents Act 1988, without the prior permission of the publisher.

Designations used by companies to distinguish their products are often claimed as trademarks. All brand names and product names used in this book are trade names, service marks, trademarks or registered trademarks of their respective owners. The publisher is not associated with any product or vendor mentioned in this book. It is sold on the understanding that the publisher is not engaged in rendering professional services. If professional advice or other expert assistance is required, the services of a competent professional should be sought.

The contents of this work are intended to further general scientific research, understanding, and discussion only and are not intended and should not be relied upon as recommending or promoting a specific method, diagnosis, or treatment by health science practitioners for any particular patient. The publisher and the author make no representations or warranties with respect to the accuracy or completeness of the contents of this work and specifically disclaim all warranties, including without limitation any implied warranties of fitness for a particular purpose. In view of ongoing research, equipment modifications, changes in governmental regulations, and the constant flow of information relating to the use of medicines, equipment, and devices, the reader is urged to review and evaluate the information provided in the package insert or instructions for each medicine, equipment, or device for, among other things, any changes in the instructions or indication of usage and for added warnings and precautions. Readers should consult with a specialist where appropriate. The fact that an organization or Website is referred to in this work as a citation and/or a potential source of further information does not mean that the author or the publisher endorses the information the organization or Website may provide or recommendations it may make. Further, readers should be aware that Internet Websites listed in this work may have changed or disappeared between when this work was written and when it is read. No warranty may be created or extended by any promotional statements for this work. Neither the publisher nor the author shall be liable for any damages arising herefrom.

*Library of Congress Cataloging-in-Publication Data*

ABC of anxiety and depression / [edited by] Linda Gask, Carolyn Chew-Graham.
  p. ; cm.
 Includes bibliographical references and index.
 ISBN 978-1-118-78079-4 (pbk.)
I. Gask, Linda, editor.   II. Chew-Graham, Carolyn, editor.
 [DNLM: 1. Depression.  2. Anxiety.   WM 171.5]
 RC537
 616.85′27–dc23

                        2014020553

A catalogue record for this book is available from the British Library.

Wiley also publishes its books in a variety of electronic formats. Some content that appears in print may not be available in electronic books.

Set in 9.25/12pt Minion by SPi Publisher Services, Pondicherry, India
Printed and bound in Malaysia by Vivar Printing Sdn Bhd

1   2014

# Contents

# Contributors

**Sarah Alderson**

Leeds Institute of Health Sciences, University of Leeds, Leeds, UK

**Clare Baguley**

Six Degrees Social Enterprise CIC, The Angel Centre, Salford, UK

**Richard Byng**

Primary Care Group, Institute of Health Services Research, Plymouth University Peninsula School of Medicine and Dentistry, University of Plymouth, Plymouth, UK

**Carolyn Chew-Graham**

Research Institute, Primary Care and Health Sciences and National School for Primary Care Research, Keele University, Keele, UK

**Jody Comiskey**

Six Degrees Social Enterprise CIC, The Angel Centre, Salford, UK

**Ceri Dornan**

Honorary Secretary, UK Balint Society; email. contact@balint.co.uk

**Chloe Preston**

Six Degrees Social Enterprise CIC, The Angel Centre, Salford, UK

**Judith Forrest**

Derbyshire Healthcare NHS Foundation Trust, UK

**Linda Gask**

University of Manchester, Manchester, UK

**Carol Henshaw**

Liverpool Women's NHS Foundation Trust, Crown Street, Liverpool, UK

**Allan House**

Leeds Institute of Health Sciences, University of Leeds, Leeds, UK

**Louise Ivinson**

Scottish Association of Psychoanalytical Psychotherapists/British Psychoanalytic Council, 19–23 Wedmore Street, London, UK

**Cornelius Katona**

Department of Psychiatry, University College London, London, UK

**David Kessler**

School of Social and Community Medicine, University of Bristol, Bristol, UK

**R. Hamish McAllister-Williams**

Institute of Neuroscience, Newcastle University, Newcastle upon Tyne, UK

**James Patterson**

Greenmoss Medical Centre, Scholar Green, Stoke on Trent, UK

**Jane Roberts**

Clinical Innovation and Research Centre, Royal College of General Practitioners, London, UK

**Aaron Vallance**

Metabolic and Clinical Trials Unit, Department of Mental Health Sciences, The Royal Free Hospital, London, UK

**Waquas Waheed**

National School for Primary Care Research, University of Manchester, Manchester, UK

**Sarah Yates**

Institute of Neuroscience, Newcastle University, Newcastle upon Tyne, UK

# Preface

We hope this book will be a useful resource for anyone who is interested in the management of common mental health problems in the primary care setting. Anxiety and depression are common and often overlap, and patients who suffer from these symptoms are usually managed in primary care.

We have drawn on our clinical experience, working in primary and secondary care, and across the interface. We have used 'cases' of fictitious characters interlinked by living in one street to illustrate the breadth of problems under the umbrella of 'anxiety and depression', reflecting our professional experiences. We hope that this makes the book appealing to a broad range of readers, including students of health and social care professions, general practitioners and primary care nurses, and practitioners working in specialist care and the voluntary (or 'third') sector.

Above all, we would like this text to contribute to an improvement in the care of people with anxiety and depression in the future.

Linda Gask
Carolyn Chew-Graham

# Acknowledgements

We thank our husbands for their patience and support, our colleagues who have contributed the chapters, and our patients whose problems inspired the 'cases'.

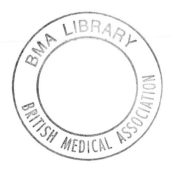

BMA LIBRARY
BRITISH MEDICAL ASSOCIATION

# List of Abbreviations

| | | | |
|---|---|---|---|
| ACE | Addenbrooke's Cognitive Examination | 5-HT | 5-hydroxytryptamine (serotonin) |
| AMTS | Abbreviated Mental Test Score | IAPT | Improving Access to Psychological Therapies |
| BA | behavioural activation | ICD | International Classification of Diseases |
| BDI | Beck Depression Inventory | 'IP' | 'in possession' |
| BME | British Minority Ethnic | LTC | long-term condition |
| CAMHS | Child and Adolescent Mental Health Services | MI | myocardial infarction |
| CBT | cognitive-behavioural therapy | MOCA | Montreal Cognitive Assessment |
| cCBT | computerised CBT | NaSSA | noradrenergic and specific serotonergic antagonist |
| CEMD | Confidential Enquiry into Maternal Deaths | NCT | National Childbirth Trust |
| COPD | chronic obstructive pulmonary disease | NHA | National Health Service |
| DBT | dialectical behaviour therapy | NSAID | non-steroidal anti-inflammatory drug |
| DSM | Diagnostic and Statistical Manual | OCD | obsessive-compulsive disorder |
| ECT | electroconvulsive therapy | PHQ-9 | Patient Health Questionnaire 9 |
| ED | Emergency Department | PTSD | post-traumatic stress disorder |
| EMDR | eye movement desensitisation reprocessing | PWP | psychological wellbeing practitioner |
| EPDS | Edinburgh Postnatal Depression Scale | QoF | Quality and Outcomes Framework |
| ESA | Employment Support Allowance | RCT | randomised controlled trial |
| FBC | full blood count | SNRI | serotonin and noradrenaline reuptake inhibitor |
| GAD | generalised anxiety disorder | SSRI | selective serotonin reuptake inhibitor |
| GP | General Practitioner | TCA | tricyclic antidepressant |
| HADS | Hospital Depression and Anxiety Scale | U&E | urea and electrolytes |
| HPA | hypothalamic-pituitary-adrenal | WHO | World Health Organization |

# CHAPTER 1

# Introduction: Anxiety and Depression

*Linda Gask[1] and Carolyn Chew-Graham[2]*

[1] University of Manchester, Manchester, UK
[2] Research Institute, Primary Care and Health Sciences and National School for Primary Care Research, Keele University, Keele, UK

Anxiety and depression are both *common mental health disorders.* They are the commonest mental health problems in the community, and the great majority of people who experience these problems will be treated in primary care.

In the UK, primary care services are an integral part of the National Health Service (NHS) in which general practitioners (GPs) work as independent contractors. The GP works as a generalist and a provider of personal, primary and continuing care to individuals, families and a practice population, irrespective of age, gender, ethnicity and problems presented.

In this book we will consider both depression and anxiety with reference to specific case histories: the O'Sullivan family and their neighbours (see Box 1.1). We will be adopting a life cycle perspective, considering depression and anxiety at different ages and times of life and in different settings although primarily taking a primary care perspective.

Box 1.1 **Broad Street**

The O'Sullivans live in a three-storey Victorian house in need of repair, in a northern English city. The extended family consists of Maria, 53, who is married to Ged; her parents, Bridie and Anthony; and Maria and Ged's sons, Patrick, 18, Francis, 20, and John-Paul, 23. Maria's brother, Frank, killed himself 10 years ago, and Bridie says she has 'never recovered'. Maria's other siblings live in Dublin, Cork and Australia.

Next door, at number 64, live the Jairaths, who also fill their house. Imran and Shabila are second-generation Pakistanis, who speak good English and both work: Imran is a businessman, importing textiles, and Shabila is a teaching assistant. Imran's parents, Hanif and Robina are in their late 70s and go out very little. Both have diabetes and Hanif had a heart attack 3 years ago, which left him anxious about his health. Shabila's four sons and one daughter, Humah, all attend the local school and seem to be doing well. The eldest son, Shochin, aged 17, is hoping to apply to study medicine. All the children attend the mosque for weekly instruction in Islam.

Number 60 is a multi-occupancy house with students who attend the local University. Jess is 19 and lives with her boyfriend, Oliver. Jess is friendly with Shabila and often looks after the younger children. She

feels she has got to know Humah, Shabila's 15-year-old daughter, quite well. Hannah has lived in the house for 2 years, and recently separated from a boyfriend. Mark and George share the top flat, and are accused by their housemates and Ged of being noisy and 'drunk'. Maria thinks they use drugs and worries about their influence on her sons.

John lives alone at number 63. He took voluntary redundancy as a supermarket manager 18 months ago. He has little to do with his neighbours. Two months after finishing work his widowed father, who lives a couple of miles away, had a stroke and John spent the next 6 months supporting his father in his recovery. John now finds himself feeling depressed, without motivation and reluctant to leave his house. He is finding it difficult to sleep. He lays awake and worries. He has stopped seeing friends, and is reluctant to talk to anyone as he thinks he has no right to feel depressed and he is a failure.

Nirma and Naeem live at number 65. Nirma is British born, 23 years old and works part time in a bank. She first saw her husband, Naeem, when she was aged 17 and on the day of her marriage (which her father had told her would be her engagement party). Her husband arrived from Bangladesh and there were no problems in the first 2 years of marriage. Then Nirma was devastated to discover that Naeem was having an affair and decided that she would leave him, although she was frightened and unsure how she would look after her two young children. Her family, who live in the next street, were not supportive of this decision, saying that this could hinder the marriage prospects of her three younger sisters. So, she remains with him, but feels her husband criticises her appearance and behaviour. She knows that he discloses their personal problems to others, which is humiliating for Nirma. Naeem is also unpredictably violent and has started to hit her in front of the children.

## What is depression?

Some people may describe themselves as 'depressed' when they are unhappy. 'Depression' is more than unhappiness: A person who is depressed will experience *low mood*, which is lower than simply being 'sad' or 'unhappy', and crucially is associated with difficulty in being able to function as effectively as is usual for them in their everyday life. The severity of this mood disturbance can vary between a mild degree of difference from the norm, through moderate levels of depression to severe depression, which may be then associated with abnormal or 'psychotic' experiences such as delusions and hallucinations. Low mood

*ABC of Anxiety and Depression*, First Edition. Edited by Linda Gask and Carolyn Chew-Graham.
© 2014 John Wiley & Sons, Ltd. Published 2014 by John Wiley & Sons, Ltd.

is accompanied by a wide range of other symptoms, which also need to be present in order to make the diagnosis of depression (see diagnostic criteria, Appendix 2). In bipolar disorder, episodes of depression and mania are both experienced. We will not be focusing specifically on bipolar disorder in this book but will highlight how, where and why it is important to distinguish bipolar from unipolar depression.

## What is anxiety?

Similarly, 'anxiety' is a term in common usage to describe feeling worried and fearful. People who are suffering with one or more of the anxiety disorders also experience symptoms of anxiety to a degree that it interferes with their ability to function. The central emotions at the heart of anxiety are fear and worry. You may be worried and fearful because you feel unsafe and have a sense of foreboding and uncertainty, as in generalised anxiety, or you may have a specific fear or phobia, or experience sudden crescendos of anxiety associated with physical symptoms, which are known as panic. Obsessive-compulsive disorder (OCD) and post-traumatic stress disorder (PTSD) are also included among the anxiety disorders (see Box 1.2).

### Box 1.2 **The spectrum of anxiety and depression***

| | Key symptoms |
|---|---|
| Depression[†] | Low mood |
| | Loss of interest or pleasure |
| Generalised anxiety disorder | Excessive anxiety and worry |
| Phobia | Fear of a specific object or situation that is out of proportion to the actual danger or threat |
| Panic disorder | Panic attacks (sudden, short-lived anxiety) |
| Obsessive-compulsive disorder | Presence of obsessions (unwanted intrusive thought, image or urge that repeatedly enters one's mind but is recognised as one's own thoughts) and/or compulsions (repetitive behaviours or acts that one feels driven to perform) |
| Post-traumatic stress disorder | Re-experiencing symptoms and aspects of a traumatic event |

*May occur separately or together in differing combinations.
[†]Depression can be unipolar or bipolar, and in severe depression psychotic symptoms may be present, which are mood-syntonic or consistent with depressed mood.

## How are anxiety and depression related?

Although they have traditionally been classified as separate disorders, there is a considerable overlap between anxiety and depression. The majority of people who are seen in primary care settings will have a mixture of symptoms of anxiety (with often symptoms of different anxiety disorders present) and depression, and often also physical symptoms that may be related to either or both of these, or for which there is no apparent physical cause

(and also other health problems too). People with more severe disorders who are seen in specialist settings may have a more distinct presentation of depression or one of the anxiety disorders, but even here they often coexist (see both Maria's and Francis's stories in Box 1.3 and Chapter 2). Anxiety may precede the development of depression and vice versa. The coexistence of symptoms had led some to question whether these are indeed distinct disorders.

### Box 1.3

**Maria's story**
'I've always been a worrier, I know that. My husband Ged says I'm always needing someone to tell me everything is going to be OK. He gets annoyed with me sometimes. I do worry about everything, especially my family. Sometimes I sit here in the armchair and it just feels as though something else awful is going to happen and I've no idea what it is. I just feel sweaty and shaky and my heart starts beating really fast. Then the other day in the supermarket, I just suddenly felt really dreadful, I suddenly started shaking and sweating, and I felt faint and I thought I was going to pass out. It was really scary. I felt awful when my brother killed himself, and I suppose I've been feeling worse since the problems started next door. I wish those boys would move out. I don't know what's happening to me. It's all really getting me down.'

**Francis's story**
'I had my first drink when I was 14. I used to get really anxious when I was out, so it gave me a bit of Dutch courage. I couldn't chat up girls if I hadn't had a drink. I was the life and soul of the party when I'd had a drink. Then it started to get a bit out of hand, and I carried on drinking when everyone else moved on, went to college and left town. I don't get out much at the moment. I have to go out to get my cider otherwise I get a bit shaky in the morning. It calms me down. I feel very stuck now. I can't seem to move on. I've started to feel really wound up and sometimes I'm *really* low. I don't tell anyone about that. I don't want to worry my mother.'

## Diagnosis and multimorbidity

The two major diagnostic systems in use for mental disorders are the *Diagnostic and Statistical Manual* of the American Psychiatric Association (DSM), which has recently been published in its fifth edition, and the *International Classification of Diseases* (now ICD-10 with edition 11 in preparation). These differ slightly in the criteria used for diagnosis of depressive and anxiety disorders. We will describe the specific symptoms associated with each way in which they can present across the life cycle in different chapters of this book.

There has been criticism about the applicability of diagnostic criteria developed in the population of people seen in specialist settings to the way in which anxiety and depression present in the wider community and in primary care. In general, presentations in primary care are less severe, though there is considerable overlap in terms of severity with those people who present to mental health services. Primary care patients frequently present a mixture of psychological, physical and social problems, and the context of life events and medical comorbidity plays an important role in how patients experience their mental health symptoms. What is clear is that overlapping degrees of psychopathology exist along a spectrum of anxiety, depression, somatisation and substance misuse. Thus, Francis (Boxes 1.1 and 1.3) has a number of problems including anxiety, depression and alcohol dependence. This coexistence may be cross-sectional in that all these symptoms appear together at the same time, or it may be longitudinal, as one set of symptoms is followed closely in time by another. All of these may occur against a background of personality difficulty or disorder. Physical health problems, especially long-term conditions such as diabetes, coronary heart disease, chronic obstructive pulmonary disease and pain (see Chapter 6) may be complicated by depression and anxiety, which will both exacerbate the distress, pain and disability associated with physical illness and adversely affect health outcomes.

## Epidemiology of depression and anxiety

Depression is a considerable contributor to the global burden of disease, and according to the World Health Organization unipolar depression alone (not associated with episodes of mania) will be the most important cause by 2030.

Estimates of prevalence vary considerably depending on the methods used to carry out the research, and the diagnostic criteria employed. In the UK the household survey of adult psychiatric morbidity in England carried out in 2007 found that 16.2% of adults aged 16 to 64 met diagnostic criteria for at least one of the common mental health disorders in the week prior to the interview. More than half of these presented with a mixed anxiety and depressive disorder (9% of the population in the last week). The 1-week prevalence for the other common mental health disorders were 4.4% for Generalised Anxiety Disorder (GAD), 2.3% for a depressive episode, 1.4% for phobia, 1.1% for Obsessive-Compulsive Disorder (OCD) and 1.1% for Panic Disorder.

Both anxiety and depression are more common in women, with a prevalence of depression around 1.5–2.5 times greater than in men. The gender difference is even greater in the South Asian population in the UK (see Chapter 8). Depression and anxiety occur in children and young people (Chapter 2), and are more common in older people than in adults of working age (Chapter 4). In the UK household survey, men and women who were married or widowed had the lowest rates of disorder, and those who were separated or divorced the highest rates. This is probably due to both the impact of separation or divorce on a person's mental health and the impact of depression in one partner on relationships. For women, family and marital stresses may be a particularly common factor leading to the onset of mental health problems. Those living in the lowest income households in society are also more likely to have a common mental health disorder. The prevalence of depression in older people is thought to be up to 20%, and 25% in people who also have a long-term physical condition (Chapter 6).

The average age of a first episode of depression or anxiety is in the early to mid-20s, but this can occur at any time from childhood (see Chapter 2) to old age (Chapter 4). Research in this area is problematic because many people with symptoms of anxiety may not seek help. A person with obsessive-compulsive symptoms may take up to 15 years or longer to seek help. In general, the earlier problems are first experienced, the more likely they are to recur, and many people with anxiety and depression experience problems from their teenage years. Given that more than 50% of people with depression will have at least one further episode, and that for many it has a relapsing and remitting course throughout their lives, depression can itself be viewed as having many of the feature of a *chronic illness,* which has important implications for treatment and longer term management. Over time, symptoms may change in severity and in form, with more anxiety than depression or vice versa. Those people who experience symptoms of panic and agoraphobia are likely to have a chronic course, and fear and avoidance of situations in which panic might occur can lead to considerable disability and social isolation.

## What causes depression and anxiety?

A combination of biological, social and psychological factors contribute to the onset of depression and anxiety. These interact with each other to differing degrees in each individual, and it is helpful to think in terms of 'vulnerability' and 'resilience' when considering the likelihood that a person will experience symptoms if they experience stress in their lives.

Within the O'Sullivan family (Box 1.1) there is a history of mental illness and, as a general rule, the more first-degree relatives who have suffered anxiety and/or depression, the more severe a person's experience of illness will be. This will not solely be as a result of genetic factors.

### Factors contributing to vulnerability and resilience

Genetic factors are important, but there is no specific gene for 'depression' or 'anxiety'. As well as influencing vulnerability, genes also control *resilience* – a low likelihood that a person will become depressed or anxious when under stress.

Early life experience increases our vulnerability, in particular maternal separation, maternal neglect and exposure to emotional, physical or sexual abuse. There is evidence that these early experiences may have biological effects – leading to hyper-responsiveness of the hypothalamic-pituitary-adrenal (HPA) axis. Later, ageing with associated loss increases vulnerability to depression.

### Factors that trigger an episode

The major contributors are severe life events (see Maria's story, Chapter 3), which are particularly likely to precipitate depression when combined with chronic social disadvantage or lack of support. Additionally, severe physical health problems can precipitate depression or anxiety, especially if it is life-threatening or causes disability. In key research carried out 30 years ago, George Brown and his colleagues demonstrated how life events were more likely to trigger depression in women living in Camberwell, south-east London, if they had three or more children under the age of 14 living at home, no paid employment outside the home and lacked a confiding relationship with another person. Financial problems, poor housing and social isolation are key stresses that can lead to the onset of symptoms.

## Factors that influence the speed of recovery

Some social factors both trigger the onset of symptoms and delay recovery. Bereavement, particularly one that is complicated, as we will see in Chapter 7, can lead to prolonged symptoms of depression in some people. Separation and divorce, physical disability, prolonged unemployment and other life events that lead to the person experiencing a sense of being chronically 'threatened' or 'trapped', such as in a prolonged and difficult marital or family dispute, can all lead to a failure to recover. We know that females are more likely than males to experience onset of symptoms and are less likely to recover; women seem to experience a greater number of distressing life events and may feel trapped by difficult marital and family circumstances.

## Psychological theories

Freud's theory of depression linked depression with the experience of loss and prolonged mourning. It can be helpful in understanding how prolonged grief develops into depression. One of the best known recent theories of depression is the cognitive theory proposed by Beck, from which *cognitive-behavioural therapy* has developed. In early life, in response to adverse events as described above, dysfunctional and quite rigid views of the self are developed (known as schemas). Life events that seem to particularly fit with these attitudes and beliefs will later trigger anxiety and/or depression. The content of these schemas is particularly negative in depression, with negative views about the self, the world and the future, such as 'I will never be a success', 'No-one will ever like me.' In anxiety, the belief will be concerned with threat, danger and vulnerability. Behavioural theories focus more on the way in which people who are depressed reduce their activity, stop doing things that are pleasurable, and become isolated, which further prolongs their depression. In *behavioural activation* the depressed person is encouraged to act better in order to begin to feel better.

## Biological factors

The monoamine hypothesis of depression and anxiety proposes that mood disorders are caused by a deficiency of the neurotransmitters noradrenaline and serotonin at key receptor sites in the brain. The way in which most antidepressants work is by altering activity at these receptors. However, it is now clear that this is far from the whole story. Inflammatory mechanisms may also play a part in the onset and continuation of depression and alter the functioning of the HPA axis. Neuroimaging studies show a significant reduction in the volume of the hippocampus in depression, and changes in activity in several regions of the brain. How these biological factors contribute to or result from the impact of life events and experiences remains a subject of much research, but cognitive-behavioural therapy has been shown in neuroimaging studies to alter functioning in specific areas of the brain linked with anxiety and depression.

## Summary

Primary care clinicians have an important role in the detection and management of anxiety and depression in patients consulting them. The importance of listening to the patient's story and understanding the context in which people live, is vital when formulating the problem and negotiating management.

## Further reading

Gask, L., Lester, H., Kendrick, A. & Peveler, R. (2009) *Primary Care Mental Health*. RCPsych, London.
Goldberg, D. (2006) The aetiology of depression. *Psychological Medicine*, **36**: 1341–1347.
Herrman, H., Maj, M. & Sartorius, N. (2009) *Depressive Disorders*, 3rd edn. Wiley Blackwell, Chichester.
Rogers, A., Pilgrim, D. & Pecosolido, B. (eds) (2011) *The SAGE Handbook of Mental Health and Illness*. SAGE Publications Ltd.

## CHAPTER 2

# Anxiety and Depression in Children and Adolescents

*Jane Roberts*[1] *and Aaron Vallance*[2]

[1]Clinical Innovation and Research Centre, Royal College of General Practitioners, London, UK
[2]Metabolic and Clinical Trials Unit, Department of Mental Health Sciences, The Royal Free Hospital, London, UK

### OVERVIEW

- Anxiety and depression are not uncommon in children and young people, particularly those with coexisting medical problems or learning difficulties.

- The primary care consultation offers an opportunity to explore the young person's problem from their own perspective, but inclusion of a family member or carer is usually necessary.

- Anxiety and depression are risk factors for self-harm and suicide.

- The stepped care approach should be followed in the management of children and young people with anxiety and/or depression.

- Psychological therapies should be considered in the first instance, and antidepressants only initiated after assessment within specialist services.

- GPs should understand referral pathways, including how to refer for specialist care.

- The third sector offers resources to support the young person and their family, and the role of the school should be recognised.

---

Box 2.1 **Introducing Humah**

Humah, 15, lives with her extended family. She is doing well at the local school, although feels her parents' expectations put all of the siblings under pressure. She has a good circle of school friends, mostly Pakistani girls approved by her parents. She likes talking to Jess next door, when she comes over to look after her three younger brothers (although can't understand why she isn't trusted… or why her older brother Shochin isn't expected to do this). She feels her mother likes chatting with Jess; in fact she only smiles when Jess is around.

   Humah feels sad most of the time and gets upset when her father and grandparents tell her she's lucky and has a bright future. She wonders whether to share her feelings with Jess, but fears she'll laugh; Jess always seems so cheerful.

---

This chapter considers the presentation and management of anxiety and depression in children and young people, and explores the challenges clinicians face in responding to the needs of children and their families. As in adults, the two conditions are frequently comorbid, but they will be discussed in turn.

### Primary care – an opportunity to make a difference

In primary care, the consultation is an opportunity for a therapeutic encounter. However, GPs often report feeling anxious and uncertain when faced with young people experiencing emotional distress – a state that can lead to inertia or disengagement and leave the young person isolated and unsure where to turn.

   A first consultation should begin the GP showing an interest and concern, thereby reinforcing that mental health issues are taken as seriously as, say, acne or period pain. This involves attentive listening and a non-judgemental stance, displaying compassion and curiosity in the young person's story. Using natural language and a lightness of tone, appropriate and judicious use of humour can serve to minimise the formal tone that clinicians can unwittingly adopt and which young people often report as a barrier. Focusing initially on the wider psychosocial context (e.g. family, friends, education/employment, how they spend their time) not only provides information but may 'break the ice' for exploring sensitive emotional issues later on. Asking about drug and alcohol use (e.g. as counterproductive coping strategies), and sexual activity/orientation are also important, but you may sense it is more appropriate to raise this later on. Establishing rapport is important for the long term: depression and anxiety in adolescence are often persistent or recurrent. Enquire about the family's mental health history: this not only might be relevant to the young person's experience, but also may cast light on the meaning of mental illness in the family. The child may have been a young carer. Moreover, evidence shows that treating parental depression or anxiety can help the child's disorder. Humah's case reflects how depression and

---

*ABC of Anxiety and Depression*, First Edition. Edited by Linda Gask and Carolyn Chew-Graham.
© 2014 John Wiley & Sons, Ltd. Published 2014 by John Wiley & Sons, Ltd.

anxiety may afflict those across generations, as well as the importance of understanding religious/cultural perspectives.

## Depression in children and adolescents

Depression is not uncommon in young people: the 1-year global prevalence rate exceeds 4% in mid–late adolescence, with increasing preponderance in girls with age. Diagnostic criteria are as for adults, although irritability, oppositional behaviours and somatic symptoms tend to be more common, whilst functionality and enjoyment in activities can often be preserved (Box 2.2). Potential contributing factors include: genetic and personality factors; parental mental health problems, conflict and lack of warmth; previous and current life events (including loss and trauma); and physical illness. School can harbour both protective factors (e.g. routine, activity, peers), exacerbating factors (e.g. bullying, stressful peer dynamics, academic worries) and consequences (e.g. deteriorating school grades or peer relationships).

---

**Box 2.2  Humah's depression**

For months Humah has struggled to get to sleep. She wakes up throughout the night and her day often starts long before her alarm. She just about manages her school-work, but worries that her difficulty in sleeping will affect her energy, concentration and school grades; her worries go round in circles, making her insomnia even worse.

Humah does as she's told and can sometimes enjoy helping out the family or being with friends. Recently she's unusually irritable though; even little things make her snap, making her feel guilty. Sometimes she feels they're better off without her, and has fleeting thoughts of wanting to die. However, she does not think she'll do anything as it will upset her family, and fears what the community might think.

---

### What to cover in the consultation

To aid diagnosis, ask direct questions about: persistence and severity of low mood, concentration, energy, enjoyment, negative thoughts, and sleep, eating and weight patterns. Risk should be evaluated at the first appointment (see below). It is better to aim for a therapeutic consultation rather than an exhaustive one; building trust is important. Ideally book further consultations there and then, which may help the young person to feel more cared for.

### Assessing and managing risk

Assessing risk can be done sensitively; for example, start by asking about hopelessness and whether life's worth living, then eventually build up to direct questions on wanting to die and then on self-harming or suicidal ideation, intent or plan (Box 2.3). There is no evidence that asking such questions increases risk, whilst an accurate risk assessment would reduce risk.

Suicidal ideation is common at some point in adolescence, although a genuine intent to kill oneself is relatively rare. Depression is particularly associated with self-harm and suicide, although teenagers may cut themselves in the absence of psychiatric disorder.

Deliberate self-harm also commonly occurs with emotionally unstable personality traits, other features of which include feelings of emptiness, emotional volatility and relationship difficulties, whilst a history of trauma or rejection is common. What to cover when assessing risk is outlined in Box 2.3. Find out about the chronology of any cutting behaviour, triggers, exacerbating and relieving factors. Although most adolescent self-harm is not acutely associated with suicide, the long-term likelihood of eventual death by suicide (in adult years) increases 50–100-fold.

---

**Box 2.3  Assessing risk**

- What methods of self-harm (or suicide) are being used or considered?
- What is the (perceived) intent? *To relieve distress? To communicate feelings? To die?*
- Have they got any firm plans? *How, what, where?*
- Is the young person unsafe at home? *Is there abuse or bullying?*
- What protective factors are there? *What might stop them from making an attempt? (e.g. impact on family and friends, or future ambitions and hopes). Who is available for them to talk to?*

---

If you are concerned about a significant and acute risk, act promptly. Confidentiality issues need to be considered, in particular deciding at what point parents need to know, and what they are told. There is often a complex balancing act between respecting the young person's right to confidentiality and maintaining short- and long-term rapport on one hand, with needing to tell parents to prevent serious risk of harm and galvanise family support and communication on the other. Gently encouraging the young person to share details with parents is often helpful. Advise parents on keeping the home safe (e.g. securing sharps and medicine).

Make an immediate referral to CAMHS (Child and Adolescent Mental Health Services) if concerned about mental health and risk, and provide as much information as possible; the time scale of a CAMHS assessment will depend on risk severity. In emergencies, CAMHS can usually respond with a same or next-day assessment; sending the young person with their family to the Emergency Department (ED) may be required. Contact your local safeguarding clinical lead or safeguarding team immediately for child protection concerns. You can seek advice from the duty social worker, without necessarily first disclosing the child's name. Share concerns with an experienced colleague and document everything clearly.

### Therapeutic options in primary care

GPs often feel they can offer little. However NICE (2005) suggests a stepped-care approach with active monitoring as the first option, unless the young person has moderate or severe depression (NICE Guidelines 28 and 90). This represents an opportunity to build a therapeutic relationship and adopt a resilience-building approach where the skills and assets of the young person themselves, and local supports, can be better employed. With permission, contacting the school can determine what they can offer (e.g. school counsellors, nurses and access to youth workers). Learning difficulties can sometimes contribute to depression and schools are well placed to intervene.

Other resources may exist locally, including NHS or charity-sector youth counselling and support, and some primary care services have links to youth workers.

If depression persists or is moderate or severe, then consider referring to specialist CAMHS services. CAMHS may offer psychological therapy including cognitive behavioural therapy (CBT), and possibly family therapy or psychotherapy. The NICE (2005) guideline for children and young people suggests psychological therapy *before* medication is considered; however, some experts advise earlier use of medication in severe depression. In addition, particularly in the current financial climate, waiting times for specialist intervention may necessitate pragmatic clinical decisions in the best interests of the patient.

Usually antidepressant prescribing is initiated and monitored by specialist CAMHS services. NICE (2005) advises fluoxetine as the first-line medication for paediatric depression as evidence suggests it has the best risk-benefit profile; other selective serotonin reuptake inhibitors (SSRIs – e.g. sertraline, citalopram) are generally second-line. SSRIs have been associated with suicidal ideation and non-fatal acts (~4%, vs 2% in placebo groups) in paediatric studies.

Overall, the majority of adolescents recover within 1 year, with episode durations typically ranging from 2 to 9 months. There is, however, a significant risk of later relapse and/or continuation into adulthood.

## Anxiety disorders in children and adolescents

### Anxiety as a state

Anxiety is a normal experience, one powerfully shaped by evolution: its very function is to keep the individual safe. Over millennia, genes bestowing the most potent 'fight-or-flight' response are passed through the generations. Anxiety comprises emotional (e.g. distress), physiological (e.g. muscle tension), cognitive (e.g. anticipation) and behavioural (e.g. escape, avoidance) responses.

### When does anxiety become a disorder?

Disorders are defined if anxiety is excessive and/or inappropriate to context or developmental stage, causing significant distress and/or impairment. The developmental aspect is important: different childhood stages are normally associated with different fears, influenced by cognitive capacity and social development. Fears of animals, monsters and darkness are typical in younger children (e.g. 3–6 years), whilst fears of failure, rejection, performance and social situations are common in teenagers. What is considered normal in a younger child may constitute a disorder in an older child. Paralleling the development of normal fears, generalised anxiety, social phobia, agoraphobia and panic disorder usually arise in adolescence, whilst separation anxiety and simple phobias occur in younger children. The evolutionary role of anxiety may explain the high aggregate point-prevalence rate of anxiety disorders of approximately 4%. One-third have two or more anxiety disorders, and 40% have another psychiatric disorder (particularly depression).

Box 2.4 **Humah's anxiety**

For months, Humah has been mulling continually over various worries. They can be about anything. Sometimes it's her *dada's* (grandfather's) health (since the heart attack, he always complains of chest pains). Sometimes she worries that her *ami* (mother) seems unhappy. Her grades have dipped since her depression and she worries about her work. Her parents don't pressurise her, but she fears she causes them disappointment. She often feels overwhelmed, feeling shaky, tense, nauseous and butterflies; sometimes she worries she's physically unwell, like her *dada*.

Humah suffers from generalised anxiety disorder *and* depression, reflecting their strong comorbidity, possibly underpinned by a shared genetic substrate. *Generalised anxiety disorder* involves persistent and varied worries (e.g. health, family, friends, school) lasting 6+ months (Box 2.4). In contrast, *panic disorder* consists of spontaneous momentary bouts of severe anxiety occurring for more than 1 month. Its unpredictability can lead to anticipatory fears of further attacks.

*Specific* or *simple phobias* are categorised according to circumstances/objects (e.g. situational, animal, nature and blood). *Agoraphobia* involves anxiety in two of: public places, crowds, leaving home or travelling alone. *Social phobia*, defined by a disproportionate fear of judgement or ridicule (e.g. whilst performing in class, social events) often leads to avoidance, thereby reinforcing anxiety. Unlike in autistic spectrum disorder, the *capacity* to socialise is generally intact. *Social anxiety disorder in childhood* and *separation anxiety disorder* (excessive anxiety about, or separating from, attachment figures) can lead to school refusal. Avoidance behaviour is common in all these anxiety subtypes. Different subtypes probably evolved to confer additional protection against specific dangers.

### Why do children get anxiety disorders?

Family studies reveal strong associations between parental anxiety/depression and anxiety disorders in their children. Twin studies point to non-shared environmental and genetic factors: heritability is 40%; complex gene–environmental interplay is likely. Neuroimaging studies reveal reduced volume in some brain regions (e.g. the limbic system). Temperament is a risk factor, including: 'inhibited temperament' (tendency to express apprehension and autonomic reactivity in unfamiliar situations), shyness and an 'anxious-resistant' attachment style.

Environmental risk factors include: parental over-control, over-protection and rejection, and modelling of anxious behaviours. Such parenting may impede the child's development of autonomy and inner security. Chronic stressors and traumatic events are also implicated. Moreover, research shows a relationship between prenatal maternal stress and childhood anxiety, a potentially evolutionary adaptive mechanism to protect the child against environmental threats. Finally, medical conditions (e.g. asthma) that cause recurrent dyspnoea increase risk, particularly for panic disorder and separation anxiety.

## Assessment and intervention

Affected children may explicitly complain of somatic symptoms rather than frank anxiety: 79% of children presenting to primary care with non-organic recurrent abdominal pain have anxiety disorder. Distinguishing normal fears from anxiety disorder is important: evaluate the triggers, severity, impact, distress and impairment.

Differential and comorbid diagnoses include: autistic spectrum disorder, depression and post-traumatic stress disorder. Exclude medical disorders and drugs that can mimic or induce anxiety states; further investigations may be indicated. Examples include: hyperthyroidism (e.g. Graves' disease), arrhythmias (e.g. supraventricular tachycardia), phaeochromocytoma, asthma and epilepsy. Implicated drugs include: street drugs (e.g. amphetamines), pseudoephedrine and caffeine.

Referral to specialist CAMHS services may be indicated. Therapeutic guidelines can be tentatively extrapolated from NICE (2011) guidance on generalised anxiety and panic disorders in adults, where psycho-education and self-help are first steps, and followed by medication *or* CBT if necessary. CAMHS services would usually consider cognitive-behavioural strategies in the first instance, with medication added if anxiety is severe, debilitating or non-responsive. Research indicates that *combining* medication with CBT is the most effective intervention.

Cognitive-behavioural therapy comprises both cognitive (e.g. challenging negative thoughts, weighing-up evidence for-and-against, positive self-talk) and behavioural methods (e.g. relaxation exercises, exposure-and-response prevention). Family and school can help the child apply coursework in between sessions. Manuals (e.g. *Think Good, Feel Good* – see 'Further reading') can provide accessible material for clinicians, young people and families, whilst evidence also supports computerised or group CBT.

Evidence leans towards SSRI medication, particularly fluoxetine, fluvoxamine and sertraline. Medication is usually continued for 6–12 months after symptom remission. Studies do not support benzodiazepines, which can carry risks (e.g. behavioural disinhibition, dependence). There is little paediatric evidence on beta-blockers.

Overall, anxiety or depression in adolescence is associated with a 2–3 times increased risk for adult anxiety disorders. Although most children with anxiety disorder are spared it in adulthood, most adults with anxiety or depressive disorders probably had anxiety disorder as children. Continuity into adulthood may be homotypic (where the same subtype of anxiety disorder re-emerges) or heterotypic (where a different subtype occurs).

## Summary

Anxiety and depression are not uncommon in children and young people, and the primary care clinician has an important role to play in detection, and working with parents, schools and third-sector youth workers to support management of the young person.

## Further reading

Association for Young People's Health. GP Champions project. Available at: http://www.youngpeopleshealth.org.uk/5/our-work/71/gp-champions-project/ (accessed 3 May 2014).

Freer, M. (2012). The Mental Health Consultation (with a young person): A toolkit for GPs. RCGP and the Charlie Waller Trust. Available at: http://www.rcgp.org.uk/clinical-and-research/clinical-resources/youth-mental-health/youth-mental-health-resources.aspx (accessed 3 May 2014).

National Institute for Clinical Excellence (2005) Depression in children and young people: identification and management in primary, community and secondary care. National Clinical Practice Guidelines CG28. NICE, London.

National Institute for Health and Clinical Excellence (2011) Generalised anxiety disorder and panic disorder (with or without agoraphobia) in adults. National Clinical Practice Guidelines, CG113. NICE, London.

Royal College of Paediatrics and Child Health. Information and resources. Safeguarding advice. Available at: http://www.rcpch.ac.uk/child-health/standards-care/child-protection/information-and-resources/information-and-resources (accessed 3 May 2014).

Stallard, P. (2002) *Think Good, Feel Good: A Cognitive Behaviour Therapy Workbook for Children and Young People*. John Wiley & Sons, Ltd., Chichester.

# CHAPTER 3

# Anxiety and Depression in Adults

*David Kessler*[1] *and Linda Gask*[2]

[1] School of Social and Community Medicine, University of Bristol, Bristol, UK
[2] University of Manchester, Manchester, UK

---

### OVERVIEW

- People suffering from depression and anxiety often present with physical symptoms.
- In primary care patients mixed symptoms of generalised anxiety and depression are common, and some patients also show specific features of the other anxiety disorders.
- Psychological treatments are preferred by many patients, but are still not always easy to access.
- Thoughts about suicide and self-harm are common in depression and it is important to ask about such thoughts.
- The management of depression and anxiety in primary care is based around the 'stepped care model'.

---

## Anxiety and depression in adults in primary care

### Introduction

This chapter considers the principles of diagnosis and management of depression and anxiety in primary care. Depression and anxiety are predominantly primary care disorders. Most people with these disorders are managed in primary care without reference to specialist help. Both disorders are very common; the estimated point prevalence of depressive episode for adults in the UK is 2.6%; if mixed anxiety and depression is included the figure rises to 11.4%. The most widely used treatment for both disorders is antidepressant drugs; in 2012 there were more than 40 million prescription items for these drugs, and most of them were written in primary care. Psychological treatments are also effective and are preferred by many patients; access to psychological therapies from primary care has been variable, but in the last few years the Improving Access to Psychological Therapies (IAPT) service has been rolled out across England to respond to the needs of patients in primary care and support primary care services.

However, recognition and management of depression is not without its problems. Research over the last 30 years has suggested that a substantial proportion of depression goes undiagnosed in primary care. Depression and anxiety are often associated with other chronic illnesses, and physical needs may seem more pressing to both doctor and patient in the context of relatively brief consultations. Doctors

have been described as being 'not very good' at following depression treatment guidelines, and even as operating the 'inverse care law' when it comes to depression in deprived communities (which means that the availability of good medical care varies inversely with the need for it in the population served). Voices within and outside the medical profession have expressed alarm at the 'medicalisation of unhappiness' and the high volume of antidepressant prescribing. Some researchers question the effectiveness of these drugs for mild to moderate disorders, and considerable work has been done to develop psychotherapeutic alternatives to be available in primary care. IAPT has shown encouraging rates of recovery in its first three years but coverage is still limited and it is acknowledged that the service does not provide enough access to high-intensity cognitive-behavioural therapy (CBT) for patients with more severe depression.

Anxiety disorders are also prominent in primary care. There are a range of anxiety disorders, including the phobias, post-traumatic stress disorder and panic disorder. In this chapter we will concentrate on General Anxiety Disorder (GAD), which is characterised by excessive worry for at least 6 months, and will only briefly consider the other anxiety disorders. It will be noted that the emphasis on the management of the common mental disorders in primary care has been on depression rather than anxiety; the drugs most widely used to treat anxiety disorders were developed for depression. The 'Quality and Outcomes Framework' (QoF) that rewards good practice in UK primary care is based around the care of depression; anxiety is not mentioned. However, anxiety and depression are often associated, either occurring together or at different times in an individual's life-course. Anxiety disorders can be chronic and disabling, and when anxiety and depression occur together, response to treatment is poorer.

There are advantages to the care of depression and anxiety being based in primary care where the emphasis is on whole person care. GPs often know their patients, their patients' families and their social setting. They are more easily accessible to patients and perceived as less stigmatising than mental health services, and have a longitudinal and developmental perspective. They may already be involved in managing the other illnesses that are so often associated with depression.

There are limitations too. Many depressed patients fear that they may be wasting the GP's time and think that doctors have more important

---

*ABC of Anxiety and Depression*, First Edition. Edited by Linda Gask and Carolyn Chew-Graham.
© 2014 John Wiley & Sons, Ltd. Published 2014 by John Wiley & Sons, Ltd.

things to do. GPs can offer a series of consultations over time but it is much more difficult to offer longer individual sessions in primary care. The emphasis of formal psychiatric training in GP vocational training schemes has tended to be on the management of psychosis rather than being targeted at depression and anxiety. However, it is not clear how to improve GP training in the management of depression and anxiety; training GPs in the management of depression has not been demonstrated in randomised controlled trials to improve outcomes.

## Presentation of depression and anxiety

Depression and anxiety can be difficult to diagnose in primary care. Patients often present physical symptoms when they are depressed and anxious, and psychological disorders often find a somatic expression. Presenting a physical symptom to the GP provides a legitimate reason for the consultation for many patients as well as being a way of addressing concerns about possible underlying physical illness. Depression and anxiety both amplify and distort patients' fears and thoughts about their bodily symptoms. Dealing with these concerns is a complex and demanding process for GPs.

For example, when Maria, whom we met in Chapter 1, talks about her anxiety and low mood (see page 2) she does not separate the symptoms into 'psychological' and 'somatic'. Maria's story illustrates how depression, anxiety and somatic symptoms occur together. She suffers from both trait and state anxiety and gives a clear description of a panic attack. She refers at the end to her low mood. In this sense the recognition of psychological distress is not difficult. However, it is possible that agreeing such a diagnosis with Maria will be more challenging. Bodily symptoms are as prominent as psychological symptoms throughout her account. They are interwoven with each other and thoughts about her family history and external environment. Her penultimate statement, 'I don't know what's happening to me' captures her bewilderment in the face of this mix of psychological and somatic distress and environmental hardship, and gives us an idea of the GP's task. For example, it is possible that Maria might present to her GP with concerns about whether she has a serious disease, perhaps something wrong with her heart. Listed in Box 3.1 are some of the strategies that may be useful when this occurs. Engagement in treatment depends on diagnostic concordance with the patient; the labels of depression and anxiety are not much use if the patient does not agree with them.

The other group of patients in whom depression and anxiety may be 'under-recognised' is one in which these disorders are more likely to occur – those suffering from other chronic illnesses such as chronic obstructive pulmonary disease (COPD), diabetes and heart disease. In this group, psychological symptoms can be pushed into the background by what appear to be more pressing physical needs. There have been attempts to address this problem by the introduction of screening questions for depression in some of those with chronic illness. In both groups of patients GPs are particularly well placed to make a diagnosis of depression or anxiety and to place it in the context of the patient's wider life, including physical illness and other comorbidities.

Francis's story in Chapter 1 (see page 2) illustrates how depression and anxiety can be complicated by alcohol and drug use. Francis began to drink to self-medicate for his social anxiety symptoms (see below) and then became physically dependent on alcohol. Alcohol and other drugs that act as central nervous system depressants (such as benzodiazepines and opiates) will then depress mood further. It can subsequently be difficult to work out which came first, the depression or the dependence.

## Assessment

Until very recently there had been an emphasis in the Quality and Outcomes Framework (QoF) in the UK on the use of symptom scales such as the nine-item Patient Health Questionnaire (PHQ9), the Beck Depression Inventory (BDI) and the General Anxiety Disorder seven-item questionnaire (GAD7) among others, as part of the assessment of depression and anxiety. These scales are generally acceptable to patients, who often value them. They can be used to monitor and illustrate change, and they often provide a basis for discussion. However, none of these questionnaires was designed as a substitute for a wider and deeper conversation. In recognition of this the QoF for depression is now based around the idea of a 'bio-psychosocial assessment', which can include symptom scores.

### What form does a bio-psychosocial assessment take?

The bio-psychosocial assessment recognises that there are a number of factors that contribute to the onset of depression and that can maintain and prolong an episode. It also encourages GPs to ask about those areas in which recovery can take place. GPs are advised to explore the domains listed in Box 3.2.

---

**Box 3.1 Techniques for managing physical symptoms associated with psychological distress**

- Acknowledge the reality of the somatic distress as well as the importance of the underlying psychological symptoms.
- Identify serious somatic symptoms and exclude underlying physical disorder.
- Don't over-investigate; it can reinforce somatic anxiety in the long term by encouraging a pattern of presentations of somatic worry relieved by tests.
- Explore patients' perspectives, their health beliefs, and how they explain or attribute their symptoms.
- Introduce the idea that the symptoms are associated with and indeed may be caused by psychological distress.
- Begin to address the psychological distress.

---

**Box 3.2 The bio-psychosocial assessment**

- Current symptoms including duration and severity.
- Personal history of depression.
- Family history of mental illness.
- The quality of interpersonal relationships with, partner, children and/or parents.
- Living conditions.
- Social support.
- Employment and/or financial worries.
- Current or previous alcohol and substance use.
- Suicidal ideation.
- Discussion of treatment options.
- Any past experience of, and response to, treatments.

NICE (Clinical Guidelines 90 and 91) has also stressed the importance of assessing functional impairment in depression, and not relying on symptom count alone. It may not be possible to cover all these areas in depth in a single GP consultation; it is a strength of general practice that the conversation between patient and doctor can evolve over a number of consultations.

The key diagnostic features of depression and generalised anxiety disorder can be found in Boxes 3.3 and 3.4.

---

Box 3.3 **Major Depressive Episode**

- Depressed mood or a loss of interest or pleasure in daily activities for more than 2 weeks.
- Mood represents a change from the person's baseline.
- Impaired function: social, occupational, educational.
- Specific symptoms, at least five of the following nine, present nearly every day, including one of the above:
  1 depressed mood or irritable most of the day, nearly every day, as indicated by either subjective report (e.g., feels sad or empty) or observation made by others (e.g., appears tearful);
  2 decreased interest or pleasure in most activities, most of each day;
  3 significant weight change (5%) or change in appetite;
  4 change in sleep – insomnia or hypersomnia;
  5 change in activity – psychomotor agitation or retardation;
  6 fatigue or loss of energy;
  7 guilt/worthlessness – feelings of worthlessness or excessive or inappropriate guilt;
  8 concentration – diminished ability to think or concentrate, or more indecisiveness;
  9 suicidality – thoughts of death or suicide, or has suicide plan.

---

Box 3.4 **Generalised Anxiety Disorder**

1 Excessive anxiety and worry occurring more days than not for at least 6 months, about a number of events or activities.
2 The person finds it difficult to control the worry.
3 The anxiety and worry are associated with three (or more) of the following six symptoms (with at least some symptoms present for more days than not for the past 6 months):
  - restlessness or feeling keyed up or on edge;
  - being easily fatigued;
  - difficulty concentrating or mind going blank;
  - irritability;
  - muscle tension;
  - sleep disturbance (difficulty falling or staying asleep, or restless unsatisfying sleep).
4 The anxiety, worry or physical symptoms cause clinically significant distress or impairment in social, occupational or other important areas of functioning.
5 The disturbance is not due to the direct physiological effects of a substance (e.g., a drug of abuse, a medication) or a general medical condition (e.g., hyperthyroidism) and does not occur exclusively during a Mood Disorder, a Psychotic Disorder or a Pervasive Developmental Disorder.

## Other common mental disorders

In primary care patients, mixed symptoms of generalised anxiety and depression are common, and some patients also show specific features of the other anxiety disorders. Patients with purer forms of the specific anxiety disorders (presenting, e.g., as panic disorder or obsessive-compulsive disorder alone without a mixture of many different anxiety symptoms) tend to have more severe symptoms and are more likely to be seen in specialist settings than in primary care. Panic attacks (see Box 3.5) may commonly occur in a person who also has depression and/or anxiety and/or symptoms of agoraphobia (see Box 3.6) but *panic disorder*, in which the panic attacks are the primary symptom, is less common. Simple phobias are common in the community and are less likely to be associated with other common mental health problems than agoraphobia or social phobia are (see Box 3.6). Obsessional symptoms may also occur in the context of depression and in obsessive-compulsive disorder. Obsessions are intrusive thoughts, images or urges that are recognised to be irrational or unwanted and are usually resisted. Compulsions are repetitive behaviours or mental acts that the person feels driven to carry out. Some questions that are useful in screening for obsessive-compulsive disorder can be found in Box 3.7. In people who have experienced life-threatening trauma, symptoms of post-traumatic stress disorder (see Box 3.8) may be present, and this may also be complicated by depression and by substance misuse.

---

Box 3.5 **What is a panic attack?**

Acute development of several of the following symptoms reaching a peak within 10 minutes:
- palpitations, pounding heart or accelerated heart rate;
- sweating;
- trembling or shaking;
- sensations of shortness of breath, smothering, choking;
- chest pain or discomfort;
- nausea or abdominal distress;
- feeling dizzy, unsteady, light-headed or faint;
- derealisation (feelings of unreality) or depersonalisation (being detached from oneself);
- fear of losing control, going crazy or even dying;
- paraesthesias (numbness or tingling sensations);
- chills or hot flushes.

---

Box 3.6 **Phobias**

**Specific phobias:** persistent and unreasonable fear of a specific object or situation (e.g., heights, spiders, injections, enclosed spaces). Often start in childhood.
**Agoraphobia:** fear of being in places or situations from which escape might be difficult or rescue unavailable. May include being in crowded places, travelling, going into shops or leaving home. Most will also have experienced panic attacks, but may avoid situations where this happens, so that they are no longer present. This is called 'fear of fear'.
**Social phobia:** persistent fear of social situations, fear of humiliation or embarrassment, leading to avoidance.

Box 3.7 **Useful screening questions for obsessive-compulsive disorder (from NICE guidance)**

- Do you wash or clean a lot?
- Do you check things a lot?
- Is there any thought that keeps bothering you that you'd like to get rid of but can't?
- Do your daily activities take a long time to finish?
- Are you concerned about putting things in a special order or are you very upset by mess?
- Do these problems trouble you?

Box 3.8 **What is post-traumatic stress disorder?**

- The person has experienced a traumatic event that involved actual or threatened death or serious injury to the self or others.
- The traumatic event is persistently relived through intrusive flashbacks, vivid memories or dreams.
- There is intense distress on re-exposure to anything that reminds the person of the events leading to avoidance.
- Pervasive hyperarousal and hypervigilance to possible danger.
- There may also be emotional numbing, difficulty in remembering the details of the trauma, and feelings of detachment or estrangement from others.

## Risk assessment in depression and anxiety

Thoughts about suicide and self-harm are common in depression and it is important to ask about such thoughts as patients may be reluctant to volunteer them; they may be ashamed or fear the consequences of disclosure. Urgent referral to specialist mental health services is recommended if a person presents a substantial risk to themselves or others. Assessment of risk of suicide and self-harm is not an exact science, but if clear intent including reference to means is expressed, this should not be ignored (see Box 3.9). Associated alcohol and drug abuse and previous serious attempts should also raise concern. Given Francis's family history of suicide and use of alcohol his potential risk of suicide is increased.

Even in the absence of suicidal thinking it is worth advising patients, families and carers on how to seek help if the symptoms worsen; agitation and anxiety often increase in the early stages of treatment.

Box 3.9 **Risk assessment: useful questions**

- How do you see the future?
- Have there been times when you felt that you wanted to get away from everything?
- Sometimes when a person feels very low, they begin to feel that life isn't worth living...have you experienced those thoughts?
- How recently?
- How often?
- Are these thoughts persistent?
- How difficult or easy is it to resist them?
- Have you made any plans?
- What exactly have you considered?
- What has stopped you from carrying this out?

# The management of depression and anxiety in primary care

The management of depression and anxiety in primary care is based around the 'stepped care model'. The principle of this model is that the intervention offered should be the least intrusive and most appropriate to the level of severity (see Box 3.10). The stepped care model is useful in guiding response to different levels of severity. Specific stepped care models have been described for depression and the anxiety disorders by NICE but we will review the basic principles here.

## Step 1

Presentations of depression and anxiety in primary care can be relatively mild. An initial assessment and recognition of the symptoms by the GP is often experienced as supportive. Psycho-education includes an explanation of the links between mental experiences and physical symptoms, for example autonomic symptoms of arousal in anxiety disorders. Advice about sleep hygiene, diet and exercise, and the establishment of regular routines can be helpful. Many patients experience a sense of relief that they have been listened to, and are reassured that they are not 'going mad'.

## Step 2

It is important to offer to review even those with apparently mild symptoms within a few weeks. They may fail to improve or feel worse. In addition, it is not always appropriate to respond to an initial presentation of depression or anxiety with 'active monitoring' and psycho-education; the need for immediate treatment may be apparent. In both depression and anxiety, persistent or worsening symptoms should trigger the offer of a 'low-intensity psychological intervention'. Such interventions include access to self-help materials, often based on CBT principles. These materials are available in books or online, and there is evidence that they are more effective when supported by a professional. Improving Access to Psychological Therapies services run self-help and psycho-educational groups in many areas. Individual psychological wellbeing practitioners (PWPs) can also offer simple behavioural interventions (see Chapter 10) that may be effective at this level of severity. The routine use of antidepressants is not recommended in this group.

## Step 3

Some patients will not respond to low-intensity interventions. These include those whose depression is more severe, and can also include patients with 'subthreshold depressive symptoms' that have been present for a long period (typically at least 2 years). The term 'subthreshold symptoms' is used for those with fewer than five of the symptoms of depression. For patients in these groups, treatment with an SSRI (selective serotonin reuptake inhibitor), antidepressant or 'high-intensity' psychotherapy such as individual CBT should be considered. Treatment choice is influenced by patient preference, and in the case of CBT, by availability. There is no reason why these treatments cannot be combined.

Box 3.10 **Stepped care**

| *Focus of the intervention* | *Nature of the intervention* |
| --- | --- |
| **Stepped care for depression** | |
| **STEP 4**: Severe and complex depression; risk to life; severe self-neglect | Medication, high-intensity psychological interventions, electroconvulsive therapy, crisis service, combined treatments, multiprofessional and inpatient care |
| **STEP 3**: Persistent subthreshold depressive symptoms or mild to moderate depression with inadequate response to initial interventions; moderate and severe depression | Medication, high-intensity psychological interventions, combined treatments, collaborative care and referral for further assessment and interventions |
| **STEP 2**: Persistent subthreshold depressive symptoms; mild to moderate depression | Low-intensity psychological and psychosocial interventions, medication and referral for further assessment and interventions |
| **STEP 1**: All known and suspected presentations of depression | Assessment, support, psycho-education, active monitoring and referral for further assessment and interventions |
| **Stepped care for GAD** | |
| **STEP 4**: Complex treatment-refractory GAD and very marked functional impairment, such as self-neglect or a high risk of self-harm | Highly specialist treatment, such as complex drug and/or psychological treatment regimens; input from multi-agency teams, crisis services, day hospitals or inpatient care |
| **STEP 3**: GAD with an inadequate response to step 2 interventions or marked functional impairment | Choice of a high-intensity psychological intervention (CBT/applied relaxation) or a drug treatment |
| **STEP 2**: Diagnosed GAD that has not improved after education and active monitoring in primary care | Low-intensity psychological interventions: individual non-facilitated self-help1; individual guided self-help; and psycho-educational groups |
| **STEP 1**: All known and suspected presentations of GAD | Assessment, support, psycho-education, active monitoring and referral for further assessment and interventions |

## Step 4

A proportion of patients do not respond to either first-line antidepressants or individual psychotherapy, or to both. Those with depression and a chronic physical health problem may also require additional therapeutic input. Specialist mental health advice is important in these groups. Options include pharmacological strategies for treatment-resistant depression, such as combining antidepressants or adding additional psychotropic drugs, and direct referral for specialist mental health care for day case or inpatient care. Specialist psychological treatments such as EMDR (Eye Movement Desensitisation Reprocessing) should also be available for people with PTSD.

## Comorbidity with alcohol and drugs

For people such as Francis who misuse alcohol, it is usual to manage the alcohol misuse problem first, as this may lead to significant improvement in symptoms. If the anxiety and depression then persist for 3 or 4 weeks, treat as above.

## Continuation and relapse prevention

Depression and anxiety can both be chronic relapsing conditions. Patients who have responded to antidepressants should be encouraged to continue their medication for at least 6 months. They can be reassured that antidepressants are not addictive, but also advised about the need to withdraw under supervision to avoid a *discontinuation syndrome*. This occurs in approximately 20% of patients after abrupt withdrawal of medication that has been taken for at least 6 weeks, and is characterised by flu-like symptoms, insomnia, nausea, sensory disturbance and hyperarousal. It is more likely for drugs with a shorter half-life.

Drug treatment may be prolonged if there is a history of recurrent depression or anxiety, but must be evaluated regularly. Individual CBT should be offered to those who relapse despite antidepressants; it can be argued that it teaches skills that are of value in the long term. There is also increasing evidence that mindfulness-based cognitive therapy is of value in preventing relapse and maintaining wellbeing.

## Summary

Most depression and anxiety can be managed in primary care. People commonly present with physical symptoms, and anxiety and depression commonly occur alongside chronic physical health problems. Engagement in treatment depends on diagnostic concordance with the patient; the labels of depression and anxiety are not of much use if the patient does not agree with them. Assessment should always including checking for thoughts of suicide or self-harm. A stepped care approach to management is very useful in tailoring treatment to severity of symptoms. Both can be chronic relapsing conditions and therefore attention should be paid to relapse prevention.

## Further reading

Chew-Graham, C.A., Mullin, S., May, C.R., Hedley, S. & Cole, H. (2002) Managing depression in primary care: another example of the inverse care law? *Family Practice* **19**: 632–637.

Gilbody, S., Whitty, P., Grimshaw, J. & Thomas, R. (2003) Educational and organizational interventions to improve the management of depression in primary care. *JAMA* **289**: 3145–3151.

NICE (2011) Common mental disorders: Identification and pathways to care. Clinical Guidelines (CG 123). National Institute for Health and Clinical Excellence.

olde Hartman, T.C., Woutersen-Koch, H. & Van der Horst, H.E. (2013) Medically unexplained symptoms: evidence, guidelines, and beyond. *British Journal of General Practice* **63**: 625–626.

## Resources

Free downloadable leaflets from the Royal College of Psychiatrists available at: www.rcpsych.ac.uk/expertadvice.aspx

Depression Alliance: www.depressionalliance.org

Anxiety UK: www.anxietyuk.org.uk

# CHAPTER 4

# Anxiety and Depression in Older People

*Carolyn Chew-Graham*[1] *and Cornelius Katona*[2]

[1] Research Institute, Primary Care and Health Sciences and National School for Primary Care Research, Keele University, Keele, UK
[2] Department of Psychiatry, University College London, London, UK

---

## OVERVIEW

- Anxiety and depression are common in older people and particularly those with chronic physical health problems.
- There are patient and practitioner barriers to the recognition and management of depression and anxiety in older people.
- Anxiety and depression in older people are risk factors for suicide.
- The stepped care approach should be followed in the management of older patients with anxiety and/or depression.
- Services adopting the principles of collaborative care should be commissioned for older people with multi-morbidity, including anxiety and depression.
- GPs should understand referral pathways, including how to access specialist care.

---

### Case study: Bridie

Bridie has never got over the death of her son, Frank, 10 years ago. She doesn't know why he killed himself, although she knew he drank (but she wouldn't admit it at the time).

She now feels 'on edge' all the time and can't settle, sometimes things improve but most of the time she feels down and miserable. Her husband, Anthony, won't talk about Frank, and her daughter, Maria, seems close to tears most of the time, so Bridie feels it's best not to say anything to the family about how she is feeling.

She decides to go and see her GP to ask for a tonic – perhaps that will lift her up.

---

This chapter considers the presentation and management of anxiety and depression in older people, and explores the challenges clinicians face in responding to the needs of older people with these common mental health problems. Depression severe enough to warrant intervention is one of the commonest mental health problems facing older people, affecting more than 1 in 10 older people in the community. There are a number of risk factors for depression, which the GP needs to be aware of (Box 4.1), and some of these are also risk factors for anxiety, particularly chronic physical conditions and loneliness.

### Box 4.1 Risk factors for depression in older people

**Physical factors**
- Chronic disease: diabetes, ischaemic heart disease, chronic obstructive pulmonary disease, inflammatory arthritides.
- Organic brain disease: dementia, Parkinson's disease, cerebrovascular disease.
- Endocrine/metabolic disorders: hypothyroidism, hypercalcaemia.
- Malignancy.
- Chronic pain.

**Psychosocial factors**
- Social isolation.
- Loneliness.
- Being a carer.
- Loss: bereavement, income, social status.
- History of depression.
- Being in institutional care.

Depression is associated with disability, increased mortality, including from suicide, poorer outcomes from physical illness, and increased use of primary and secondary and social care resources. Major depression is a recurring disorder and older people are more at risk of recurrence than the younger population.

Anxiety disorders are also common in older people. 'Anxiety' covers the terms generalised anxiety disorder (GAD), panic and phobic disorders. GAD is a common disorder, of which the central feature is excessive worry about a number of different events associated with heightened tension. Anxiety and depression often coexist (or overlap) in older people and may also be comorbid with physical conditions (leading to poorer outcomes in those conditions).

Patients with anxiety disorders may complain of worry, irritability, tension, tiredness or 'nerves', but older people may present with somatic symptoms that may cause diagnostic difficulty for the GP and (if not identified) may result in unnecessary investigations for the patient – with the resultant worries aggravating the depression and anxiety symptoms. The GP needs to be aware of the link with alcohol misuse and should always explore alcohol consumption in older people who present with symptoms of depression or anxiety.

---

*ABC of Anxiety and Depression*, First Edition. Edited by Linda Gask and Carolyn Chew-Graham.
© 2014 John Wiley & Sons, Ltd. Published 2014 by John Wiley & Sons, Ltd.

Older people consult their primary care practitioner more frequently than younger people, and those who are depressed consult twice as often as those who are not. Despite this, depression is diagnosed less often in older people. Older people who are depressed can present with nonspecific symptoms rather than disclosing depressive symptoms. Standard diagnostic criteria (ICD 10, DSM – for anxiety and depression) have been developed to reflect symptoms observed in younger people. They have inherent limitations for diagnosis of depression in older people, whose presentation may differ because of ageing, physical illness or both. Other clinical features often found in older people include: somatic preoccupation, hypochondriasis and the morbid fear of illness, which are more common presentations than the complaint of low mood or sadness. In addition, physical symptoms, in particular seemingly disproportionate pain, are common and the primary care clinician may feel they represent organic disease. This can cause problems for the GP, as a depressed patient's hypochondriacal complaints can be quite different from the bodily symptoms one might expect from knowledge of the patient's medical history. Subjective memory disturbance may be a prominent symptom and lead to a differential diagnosis of dementia, but true cognitive disturbance is also common in late-life depression. The GP should assess memory using the GPCOG (see 'Resources' below) or the Abbreviated Mental Test Score (see Appendix 4).

Depression in older people (particularly when there is no history of depression earlier in the patient's life) is associated with increased risk of subsequently developing a 'true' dementia. Lastly, a persistent complaint of loneliness in an older person (even when that person is known to live with others) should prompt enquiry into mood, feelings, views on the future, and a more systematic enquiry about biological symptoms of depression, along with a formal assessment, including a risk assessment.

Older adults may have beliefs that prevent them from seeking help for mental health problems, such as a fear of stigmatisation or concern that antidepressant medication is addictive. They may not consider themselves candidates for care because of previous experience of help-seeking. In addition, older people may be reluctant to recognise and name 'depression' as a specific condition that legitimises attending their GP, or they may misattribute symptoms of major depression for 'old age', ill health or grief and use normalising attributional styles that see their depression as a normal consequence of ill health, of difficult personal circumstances or even of old age itself. GPs may lack the necessary consultation skills and confidence to correctly diagnose depression in older people, and anxiety is particularly under-diagnosed. They may also be wary of opening a 'Pandora's box' in time-limited consultations and instead collude with the patient in what has been called 'therapeutic nihilism'. Additionally, a lack of congruence between patients' and professionals' conceptual language about mental health problems, along with deficits in communication skills on the part of both patients and professionals, can lead to uncertainty about the nature of the problem and reduce opportunities to talk about appropriate management strategies.

The use of case-finding questions (Box 4.2) should be part of usual practice for GPs in consultations with older people who have

---

**Case study: Bridie (cont'd)**

Bridie tells the GP that she feels tired all the time and is not sure what is wrong. The GP suggests some blood tests and she leaves the practice with instructions to make an appointment with a healthcare assistant. She is not quite sure why she didn't mention how upset she feels. She decides to make an appointment with a different GP whom she has seen before and who, she thinks, will give her more time and invite her to talk about how she feels.

---

Box 4.2 **Case-finding questions**

During the past month, have you often been bothered by feeling down, depressed or hopeless?
During the past month, have you often been bothered by having little interest or pleasure in doing things?
A 'yes' to either question is considered a positive test. A 'no' response to both questions makes depression highly unlikely.

---

risk factors for depression and anxiety (Box 4.1) or where the GP has a clinical suspicion that depression may be present. The questions should be used as prompts by the GP, rather than formal 'screening' questions whose wording has to be adhered to rigidly.

The GP should cover five areas in the primary care consultation when anxiety and/or depression are suspected in an older person: history, mental state, risk assessment, focused physical examination and appropriate investigations. The latter should include full blood count (FBC), urea and electrolytes (U&Es), liver and thyroid function tests, vitamin $B_{12}$ and folate, glycosylated haemoglobin (HbA1C), bone profile and any further tests dictated by clinical presentation. It is particularly important to establish risk of self-harm. This is often overlooked when the predominant symptom is anxiety, but older patients are at risk of self-harm and self-neglect, and the GP should be aware of this. GPs may shy away from asking about suicide for fear of 'putting thoughts into the patient's head'. Providing an opportunity to disclose suicidal thoughts or plans may, on the contrary, be a huge relief for patients who may until then have felt ashamed of these thoughts and fearful of disclosing them. Assessment of severity of anxiety (using GAD-7 – see Appendix 1) and depression (PHQ-9 – see Appendix 2) should be considered in order to contribute to the management plan.

Some clinicians consider anxiety and depression to be part of a continuum and that the overlap between them is particularly broad in older people. Labelling the patient as having one disorder or the other may be less important than assessing the severity and impact of the mood disorder on the patient's life. This may be a valid perspective in primary care, where people often present with mixed or comorbid problems, but it is important to distinguish which symptoms are most prominent in order to focus explanations and identify appropriate management options. It is vital that the GP explores the patient's ideas and concerns about their problem, and the expectations the patient may have of both the GP and of any treatment offered. Any explanation given by the GP needs to fit with the patient's model of their problem. This can require considerable skill and cultural sensitivity on the part of the GP, and may require a number of consultations before an older person is willing to consider 'anxiety' or 'depression' as a working diagnosis on which to base a management plan.

For both anxiety and depression, the 'stepped care model' provides a framework in which to plan individual patient management. The NICE guidelines for anxiety and depression (National Collaborating Centre for Mental Health, 2010 and 2009) offer a stepped care model for the management of people with anxiety, and this approach is appropriate for older people with anxiety symptoms, with or without depression. Thus, discussion with the patient about the symptoms and their meaning should occur, followed by negotiation of a management plan acceptable to the patient. When physical symptoms are the presenting problem, appropriate physical examination may help to reassure the patient that their symptoms are being taken seriously, but repeated investigations should be avoided. Initial management should involve verbal and written information about anxiety, signposting to age-appropriate support groups (e.g. Age UK) or self-help groups (Anxiety UK), and discussion of behavioural activation (BA) techniques (see Chapter 10), with an arrangement to follow the patient up. Appropriate advice about alcohol and physical activity as in the management of depression should be given. A similar approach should be taken when depressive symptoms are predominant.

If there is no improvement of symptoms following such 'active monitoring' and support from the GP and referral to third sector services, then discussion with the patient about the acceptability of referral for 'low-intensity psychological interventions' should take place. There is evidence that older people are less likely to be referred for CBT-based interventions, despite the fact that the evidence base for their use is similarly good for older people and for adults of working age. If a 'talking treatment' is unacceptable to the patient, then the GP should discuss how the patient would feel about taking antidepressants and the rationale for this suggestion.

Management of anxiety and depression in older people should follow that suggested by national guidelines and be no different to that in younger adults, although the likelihood of comorbid physical health problems means that a collaborative care approach may be particularly indicated (Box 4.3).

---

Box 4.3 **Components of the Collaborative Care framework***

A multi-professional approach to patient care delivered by a GP and at least one other health professional (e.g., a nurse, psychologist, psychiatrist or pharmacist).
A structured patient management plan that facilitates delivery of evidence-based interventions (either pharmacological or 'talking treatments').
Scheduled and proactive patient follow-ups, either face-to-face or by remote communication (e.g., telephone).
Enhanced inter-professional communication between team members who share responsibility for the care of the patient (e.g., team meetings, case conferences, supervision).

*See Gunn et al. (2006) under 'Further reading' below.

---

It is important that GPs are aware of the service offered by their local primary care mental health team, and by local IAPT (Improving Access to Psychological Therapies) services. They should ensure that a range of evidence-based services for all patient groups (specifically including older people) are commissioned by their Clinical Commissioning Groups.

SSRIs are the first-line antidepressants for older people with depression or anxiety (see Chapter 11). Patients starting on SSRIs should be warned about common side effects that can occur in the first few days or weeks of treatment (such as nausea, fatigue, headache and increased anxiety), and possible longer-term side effects (such as reduced libido and weight gain). GPs should be particularly aware of the risk of gastrointestinal bleeding (particularly if the patient is taking aspirin) and hyponatraemia, both of which are commoner and potentially more dangerous in older people. The patient should be warned about the 'withdrawal' side effects of stopping an antidepressant abruptly and that it is vital to continue the antidepressant for at least 9 months (longer if this is an episode of recurrent depression). Should an SSRI be ineffective, second-line antidepressants the GP might wish to prescribe include mirtazapine or venlafaxine. Such prescribing decisions need to take account of relevant comorbidities such as cardiovascular disease and of potential drug interactions.

Even if the GP has referred a patient to another service, and especially if the patient has agreed to take an antidepressant, active follow-up and monitoring of the patient is required. The GP can use basic BA techniques, even in a time-limited consultation, making use of available bibliotherapy to support this. Regular review is vital to ensure risk is assessed and responded to.

---

**Case study: Bridie (cont'd)**

Bridie was initially reluctant to take the tablets that her doctor gave her and didn't see how tablets would help change the way she felt, but when she hit 'rock bottom' she thought she would give them a chance. She has tried two different sorts now, but 3 months down the line she feels no better, and is starting to feel desperate. Her husband tells her she looks ill and her grandchildren say she is becoming forgetful. Her doctor advised her to stop the glass of whisky before bed, but she is actually drinking more as that's the only way she can stop worrying and get to sleep, She is sure that the whisky makes her feel worse in the morning and is also worried the whisky might be interfering with the tablet that she has been told to take at night.

---

There are several clinically worrying features at this point. Bridie has failed to respond to two antidepressants. Her forgetfulness may be integral to her depression but may also be a presenting feature of an underlying dementia. Bridie's escalating alcohol use may well be an important 'maintenance' factor making her depression less likely to respond to treatment. It may also be contributing to her cognitive difficulties. In view of the increasingly evident complexity of her mental health difficulties and her lack of response to treatment, it would be appropriate for Bridie to be referred to the local community mental health team for older people.

If Bridie agreed to referral, she may be assessed by a community mental health nurse in the first instance. This assessment could take place either at her home or in a clinic, depending on local arrangements. The assessment would include taking a full history from Bridie herself (including her adherence to recent antidepressant treatment and her recent and longer-term alcohol intake) and, where possible, from her husband. Bridie's mood would also be assessed, probably with a rating scale designed for older people such as the Geriatric Depression Scale (GDS; see Appendix 3), as would her cognitive function (using a validated rating scale such as the Montreal Cognitive Assessment or the Addenbrooke's Cognitive Examination (ACE III) (see Appendices 7 and 8). Further investigation would include brain imaging (CT or MRI scan). Treatment should include addressing Bridie's alcohol use and 'augmenting' her antidepressant with a second antidepressant, lithium or an atypical antipsychotic. If there is significant cognitive impairment, however, antipsychotics should be avoided if at all possible. If Bridie continued to deteriorate (e.g., by refusing food or fluid or by manifesting active suicidal intent), inpatient treatment should be considered (which may have to be under the provisions of the Mental Health Act), as might treatment with electroconvulsive therapy (ECT).

## Summary

Anxiety and depression are common in older people with multi-morbidities and are risk factors for suicide. The primary care clinician has an important role in the detection and management of anxiety and depression, and should be aware of when to refer for specialist input.

## Further reading

Buszewicz, M. & Chew-Graham, C.A. (2011) Improving detection and management of anxiety disorders in primary care [invited editorial]. *British Journal of General Practice* **589**: 489–490.

Burroughs, H., Morley, M., Lovell, K., Baldwin, R., Burns, A. & Chew-Graham, C.A. (2006) 'Justifiable depression': how health professionals and patients view late-life depression; a qualitative study. *Family Practice* **23**: 369–377.

Gunn, J., Diggens, J., Hegarty, K. & Blashki, G. (2006) A systematic review of complex system interventions designed to increase recovery from depression in primary care. *BMC Health Services Research*, **6**: 88.

National Collaborating Centre for Mental Health (2009) Depression: the treatment and management of depression in adults (updated edition). National Clinical Practice Guideline 90. British Psychological Society and Royal College of Psychiatrists, Leicester and London.

National Collaborating Centre for Mental Health (2011) Generalised anxiety disorder in adults: management in primary, secondary and community care. National Clinical Guideline 113. British Psychological Society and Royal College of Psychiatrists, Leicester and London.

National Institute for Health and Clinical Excellence (2009) Depression in adults with a chronic physical health problem. NICE Clinical Guideline 91. National Collaborating Centre for Mental Health, London.

Whooley, M., Stone, B. & Sogikian, K. (2000) Randomized trial of case-finding for depression in elderly primary care patients. *Journal of General Internal Medicine* **15**: 293–300.

## Resource

GPCOG (The General Practitioner assessment of COGnition): http://www.gpcog.com.au

# CHAPTER 5

# Antenatal and Postnatal Mental Health

*Carol Henshaw[1] and James Patterson[2]*

[1] Liverpool Women's NHS Foundation Trust, Crown Street, Liverpool, UK
[2] Greenmoss Medical Centre, Scholar Green, Stoke on Trent, UK

---

### OVERVIEW

- Anxiety and depression are common complications of pregnancy and the postpartum period.
- They not only have a significant impact on maternal wellbeing but also can lead to adverse obstetric, fetal and infant outcomes.
- Case-finding and appropriate assessment are essential. Women should be referred for evidence-based management.

---

Box 5.2 **Risk factors for postnatal depression**

- Past history of depression or anxiety.
- Depression and anxiety during pregnancy.
- Life events.
- Lack of support or perceived lack of support.
- Difficult relationship with a partner.

## Background

This chapter considers what is known about anxiety and depression during pregnancy and in the postpartum period and the effective treatments. We will discuss this in relation to the two cases in Box 5.1.

---

Box 5.1 **Shabila and Hannah**

Shabila is due to deliver her sixth child in 2 weeks time. She couldn't believe she was pregnant when she found out, she had thought those days were over and was happy with her bit of independence her part-time job gave her. Her husband and his parents were pleased with the news of the pregnancy, whilst her children seemed indifferent, apart from Humah, who seems very quiet these days and seems to avoid being with the family. Lately, Shabila has felt too tired to do the housework, but she can't sleep however tired she feels. She hopes she feels different when the baby is born.

Hannah is 22 and in her final year at university. All was going well until her boyfriend decided to leave 4 months ago. She didn't tell him she was pregnant. She has managed to cope with her studies with the support of her friends on her course. Her housemates, particularly Jess, are very supportive, and have said she can stay (although they haven't told the landlord yet), but she feels increasingly isolated from her university friends, and her family, and is struggling to cope with her situation. Her parents, who live a good distance away, were shocked that she didn't consider a termination.

---

## Depression

Postnatal depression is the most common medical complication of childbirth and follows around 13% of deliveries. Higher rates are reported in areas with social adversity and deprivation. There are a number of factors that increase the risk of postnatal depression (see Box 5.2). This leaves women like Hannah – in the second case study in Box 5.1 – vulnerable to depression following delivery as her partner has left, she is feeling isolated from her friends, and her parents are disapproving of her situation. Shabila, in the first case study, feels unsupported by her children and already has some symptoms suggestive of depression, which increase her risk after delivery.

Untreated depression can last for a few weeks to a few months but around 10% of cases will last into the second year after childbirth. Pregnancy has often been thought to be a time of emotional wellbeing but depression is as common during pregnancy as it is after delivery. Up to one-third of postnatal depressive episodes have onset during pregnancy. Three to five percent of women will experience a depression severe enough to require referral to secondary mental health care, and 1 in 500 will suffer a puerperal psychosis. Two-thirds of puerperal psychoses are psychotic depressions and one-third are manic episodes. Manic episodes tend to onset more rapidly than depression but more severe depressive episodes can also develop quickly.

---

*ABC of Anxiety and Depression*, First Edition. Edited by Linda Gask and Carolyn Chew-Graham.
© 2014 John Wiley & Sons, Ltd. Published 2014 by John Wiley & Sons, Ltd.

## Anxiety

Less attention has been paid to anxiety disorders in the perinatal period, but they are as common as depression and comorbidity with depression is not unusual. Generalised anxiety disorder, panic disorder and phobic disorders occur during pregnancy and postpartum, and some women suffering from depression will experience anxiety symptoms such as panic attacks, intrusive obsessional thoughts or compulsions during a depressive episode.

Severe anxiety during pregnancy often focuses on fear of miscarriage or stillbirth (particularly if there is a history of reproductive loss) and fetal abnormality. After delivery, fears of a cot death or of being criticised as a mother are common.

Obsessional symptoms often focus on cleaning or hand washing and fears that the baby might become infected with something. Sometimes compulsive checking of the baby to make sure he or she is still breathing can occur. Some women experience distressing intrusive obsessional thoughts that some harm might come to their baby. This can be misinterpreted as intention to harm, and careful clinical assessment is essential to distinguish between obsessional thoughts that a mother is not going to carry out and a woman with thoughts of harming her child that she is at risk of acting on.

Post-traumatic stress symptoms and post-traumatic stress disorder (PTSD) can occur after traumatic deliveries. Women with a history of sexual trauma and/or mental health problems are at increased risk, but perceived poor support in labour from a partner or professionals, being in pain, perceived loss of control, feeling powerless and medical interventions are also important. It can lead to fear of future childbirth (*tokophobia*), and some women will avoid or terminate a pregnancy of a much-wanted baby, or may demand a Caesarean section as a result.

Phobic anxiety can also require assessment and intervention if it might have an impact on care during pregnancy and labour. Needle and blood phobias can be treated effectively with systematic desensitation, and if they are identified at booking for antenatal care prompt referral is essential so that treatment can start as soon as possible.

## Impact of depression and anxiety during pregnancy

Anxiety and depression during pregnancy are associated with a number of adverse obstetric outcomes (see Box 5.3).

---

**Box 5.3 Adverse obstetric outcomes associated with anxiety and depression during pregnancy**

- Pre-eclampsia.
- Increased nausea and vomiting, longer work absence during pregnancy.
- Elective Caesarean delivery and epidural analgesia during labour.
- Admission of the infant to neonatal care.

---

Depression and anxiety during pregnancy and after delivery have been associated with cognitive, emotional and behavioural problems in the child that persist throughout their school years. Boys seem to be more vulnerable to these effects, and postpartum they are thought to be mediated via disturbed mother–infant interaction. There is an also an association with sudden infant death syndrome although the mechanism for this is unknown.

## Case-finding and assessment

Many women who become depressed during pregnancy or after delivery will seek help, but not all do. Some women may not recognise themselves as being depressed or having a problem. Others may be feeling ashamed, stigmatised or fearful that their children may be removed by Social Services. Hence, case-finding for depression during pregnancy and after delivery is recommended by various guidelines including that of NICE (Clinical Guideline 45). Many pregnant or postpartum women also experience a number of symptoms similar to those of depression, particularly disturbances of sleep, appetite and energy levels. Like Shabila in the case study (Box 5.1), they might hope that things will improve but they may not, and what a woman thinks might be normal for a new mother could develop into a depressive illness.

Several different measures are available and validated to use for case-finding for depression in postpartum women. The most extensively researched is the Edinburgh Postnatal Depression Scale (EPDS; see Appendix 5), which has now been translated into over 60 different languages, but the Whooley Questions, PHQ-9 (see Appendix 2) and the Hospital Anxiety and Depression Scale (Appendix 6) are also used, and in the USA, the Postpartum Depression Screening Scale.

At all antenatal bookings, in addition to asking about current depression, women should be asked about any history of serious mental illness, puerperal psychosis, any psychiatric admission or treatment by mental health services. Mood should be monitored by midwives during pregnancy alongside physical maternal and fetal wellbeing.

Most guidelines advocate case-finding for depression on two occasions postpartum. The first coincides with the 6-week postnatal check and can be undertaken by a health visitor or GP, preferably someone who already has a good relationship with the mother and who is familiar with local referral pathways and services. As some depressive episodes onset later, case-finding at 3–4 months after delivery is advocated, but more difficult to complete as it is likely that women will have reduced contact with the health visitor, and may not consult a GP for her own health. Frequent consultations about the baby may indicate underlying anxiety or depression in the mother, and the GP needs to be sensitive to this.

Very severe depressive disorders and particularly psychotic depression can onset rapidly after delivery, especially if there is a history of severe mood disorder. The early symptoms can be quite non-specific, for example, insomnia, agitation, irritability or excess anxiety, and can be easily dismissed; but the woman can develop profound depressive symptoms with thoughts of self-harm, or psychotic symptoms. Thus, in a woman with a past history of postnatal depression, such symptoms should not be dismissed and she should be closely monitored by the GP and health visitor.

## Suicide and risk assessment

Any woman with depressive symptoms should also be asked about thoughts of harming herself or others, and a positive answer to this, or to question 10 of the EPDS – 'the thought of harming myself has occurred to me' – requires further exploration. It is necessary to establish whether she has thought of methods and made plans, or can resist the thoughts and what is stopping her carrying them out ('protective factors'). A woman who is actively suicidal or unable to resist thoughts of harming another person, including her baby, requires urgent psychiatric assessment. Postpartum women tend to use violent methods of harming themselves, such as jumping from high buildings, in front of trains, hanging or setting fire to themselves, unlike women in the general population, and are thus more likely to succeed.

It is also important to remember that postpartum women are at increased risk of some serious medical conditions. Women have died because a history of mental disorder meant that symptoms of medical disorders were attributed to their anxiety or depression and they were treated inappropriately (Confidential Enquiry into Maternal Deaths, CEMD). For example, a woman presenting with tachycardia and double incontinence was admitted to a psychiatric hospital. Although she was later transferred to an intensive care unit, she died of sepsis and cardiac arrhythmia. An acute confusional state secondary to subdural haematoma following a fall in a woman with alcohol problems was attributed to depression, and a woman presenting with anxiety accompanying severe upper back pain was diagnosed as suffering from postnatal depression even when she went on to complain of shortness of breath, chest pain and haemoptysis. She was agitated and frightened of dying and later died of pulmonary embolism and aortic dissection.

## Interventions

Women with mild disorders can benefit from guided self-help and an introduction to local support groups, or telephone or online support. Health visitors trained in non-directive counselling or cognitive-behavioural skills can effectively support women with mild to moderate depression.

Those with moderately severe depression can benefit from psychological therapies such as cognitive-behavioural therapy or interpersonal therapy. This can be delivered on an individual or group basis, and access to such therapies has improved with the IAPT initiative in England. Such referrals should be accepted as priority cases by these services.

In women with moderate to severe depression and/or anxiety, antidepressants are indicated. The GP needs to sensitively suggest the need for antidepressants and explore the woman's views on medication. Women may be reluctant to consider tablets, particularly if they are breast feeding, and need reassurance that antidepressants are safe when breastfeeding. Hannah has been looking at a number of unreliable internet sources and says she would not take antidepressants while pregnant or breastfeeding because they might harm her baby. Health professionals counselling women who need medication while pregnant or breastfeeding should be aware of the resources available to assist in providing accurate evidence-based information so that they can advise women appropriately (see 'Further reading').

Signposting women to third sector services, the National Childbirth Trust (NCT) and online support groups can be helpful for women to appreciate that they are not alone. This might be helpful for women like Shabila who could miss the independence and social contact of her job while on maternity leave and not feel supported by her older children. Hannah, who no longer has a partner and lacks support from those around her, would probably also benefit from other forms of support, and an awareness by the GP of third sector support is important.

Women who suffer from severe depression who are actively suicidal and/or have psychotic symptoms such as delusions and hallucinations are likely to require inpatient care. Those with such problems who are in late pregnancy or postpartum should be admitted to a specialist mother and baby unit (with their baby if postpartum). Such units are best placed to treat severe perinatal mood disorders and maintain the mother-infant relationship. However, they are not present in all cities, and large parts of the UK (including all of Wales and Northern Ireland) have none at all, so this may mean admission at some distance from home. Most units have specialist community teams attached who can facilitate early discharge as soon as this is appropriate and support women at home who do not require admission.

## Summary

Depression and anxiety occurring during pregnancy or after childbirth not only cause distress for the woman concerned but also can have an adverse impact on the pregnancy and baby. Hence it is important that such women are identified and fully assessed, and that appropriate and effective treatment are offered depending on the severity of the disorder. Professionals in contact with pregnant or postpartum women must be familiar with their local care pathways and services.

## Further reading

Alder, J., Fink, N., Bitzer, J., Hösli, I. & Holzgreve, W. (2007) Depression and anxiety during pregnancy: A risk factor for obstetric, fetal and neonatal outcome? A critical review of the literature. *Journal of Maternal-Fetal and Neonatal Medicine* 20: 189–209.

Brockington, I.F., Macdonald, E. & Wainscott, G. (2006) Anxiety, obsessions and morbid preoccupations in pregnancy. *Archives of Women's Mental Health* 8:253–263.

Cantwell, R., Cluttton-Brook, T., Cooper, G. *et al.* (2011) Saving Mothers' Lives: Reviewing maternal deaths to make motherhood safer: 2006–2008. The Eighth Report of the Confidential Enquiries into Maternal Deaths in the United Kingdom. *British Journal of Obstetrics and Gynaecology* 118(S1): 1–203.

Cox, J., Holden, J. & Henshaw, C. (2014) *Perinatal Mental Health: The Edinburgh Postnatal Depression Scale Manual*, 2nd edn. RCPsych Publications, London.

National Institute for Health and Clinical Excellence (2007) Antenatal and postnatal mental health: clinical management and service guidance. National Clinical Practice Guideline Number 45. Available at: http://www.nice.org.uk/CG045fullguideline (accessed 3 May 2014).

Scottish Intercollegiate Guideline Network (2012) Management of perinatal mood disorders. A National Clinical Guideline SIGN 127. Available at: http://www.sign.ac.uk/pdf/sign127.pdf (accessed 3 May 2014).

Williams, C., Cantwell, R. & Robertson, K. (2008) *Overcoming Postnatal Depression: A Five Areas Approach*. Hodder Arnold, London.

## Advice on prescribing

National Poisons Information Service. Toxbase: http://www.toxbase.org/ [for health professionals and requires registration].

UK Teratology Information Service: http://www.uktis.org/ [patient information leaflets coming soon].

# CHAPTER 6

# Anxiety and Depression: Long-Term Conditions

*Sarah Alderson and Allan House*

Leeds Institute of Health Sciences, University of Leeds, Leeds, UK

## OVERVIEW

- Patients with long-term conditions have a high prevalence of comorbid depression and anxiety.
- Presentation of anxiety and depression in people with long-term conditions (LTCs) can by atypical.
- Causes of anxiety and depression include societal factors and other negative life events, as well as the long-term condition.
- Patient, professional, organisational and societal factors are barriers to effective diagnosis and management of anxiety and depression in LTCs.
- The management of depression and anxiety in patients with long-term conditions may be improved through the adoption of common principles of 'chronic disease management' and 'collaborative care'.

Depression and anxiety are common in people who have long-term physical conditions (LTCs) and can be more difficult to detect and treat. Less attention has been given to anxiety, but anxiety and depression often coexist, and mixed presentations are common in primary care. Anxiety symptoms can have significant overlap with those of the physical illness, particularly chest pain in those with cardiac disease and shortness of breath in chronic obstructive pulmonary disease (COPD) and asthma.

### Case study: Hanif

Hanif is 78 years old and came to England 40 years ago. He set up a business and was proud to buy number 60 Broad Street. He has had diabetes for at least 20 years, and wasn't surprised to be told he had this condition as it seems everyone in his family eventually gets it. He tries to follow a diet and does take his tablets, unlike his wife who was diagnosed about 14 years ago and doesn't seem to bother. He was so angry when it was he who had a heart attack 4 years ago – it just came out of the blue when he was digging in the garden. The hospital staff were wonderful, but after he was sent home, he felt no one really bothered about him, and since then he has been so worried about what he can and can't do. His wife accuses him of being lazy and his son tells him he is OK. Only his grand-daughter, Humah, seems to care for him; she is always so attentive and sits with him when he gets upset.

## The nature of the problem

Hanif's symptoms – anger, worry, getting upset – indicate an emotional response to his illness that is associated with family tensions. Could he have a significant mood disorder? Depression can be difficult to recognise in the presence of long-term physical conditions – because there is overlap of physical symptoms such as lethargy or poor sleep; the presenting symptoms of depression are varied and not clearly defined, and patients may be reluctant to talk about emotional problems with healthcare professionals.

Hanif's non-specific symptoms should be followed up with more specific inquiry about his mood, since he is functionally impaired by his emotional state and is fearful of activity rather than being limited solely by his heart disease. Case-finding questions can help identify depression in people with LTCs, but need to be supplemented with clinical judgement as, if used alone, they overestimate the presence of coexisting depression.

Depression associated with long-term conditions is associated with a significant increase in morbidity and mortality (Box 6.1). The best evidence is in conditions such as cardiac disease and diabetes, but the risks are present in any chronic condition such as psoriasis, chronic pain and COPD. There may be physiological explanations for this comorbidity – chronic depression is associated with a persistent endocrine stress response and with a low-grade inflammatory response – but more immediately relevant clinically are factors such as reduced adherence to treatment, poor diet, misuse of alcohol and limited physical activity – all exacerbated by depression. Similarly, comorbid depression can lead to poor medication adherence, difficulties in self-management and reduced physical activity (Box 6.1).

People with comorbid depression and anxiety can present with functional impairment that appears to be out of proportion to the clinical severity of physical illness, and case identification should take into account not just 'symptom count' but the severity of emotionally related disability.

*ABC of Anxiety and Depression*, First Edition. Edited by Linda Gask and Carolyn Chew-Graham.
© 2014 John Wiley & Sons, Ltd. Published 2014 by John Wiley & Sons, Ltd.

Box 6.1 **Consequences of comorbid anxiety and depression**

- Reduced adherence to treatment.
- Increased unplanned hospital admissions.
- Increased healthcare costs.
- Lower quality of life.
- Increased morbidity.
- Increased mortality.

## Theories about aetiology

People with chronic illness also suffer the same losses, role changes and stresses as the normal population, and not all anxiety and depression will be related to the physical condition. Even so, the prevalence of mood disorder in physical illness is two to three times that in the general population. This higher prevalence is usually attributed to the specific meaning for the individual and impact upon their life of the long-term condition, which may represent *a threat* that causes anxiety or anger and irritability in response to uncertain risk; *a sense of loss* for the future self, which includes facing mortality and disability; a *lack of personal control* over what is happening; and *humiliation* over the loss of position in society or family and undermining the sense of self. The psychological challenges posed by illnesses may lead to depression or anxiety if the individual is not able to mount an effective coping response.

Professional views on the causes of depression associated with LTCs tend to emphasise poor coping with the challenges of the illness, increased vulnerability and poor social support. However, patients do not necessarily understand their distress as a discrete state that might be diagnosed, labelled and treated. They may be reluctant to admit their distress or fear stigmatising responses from others (including healthcare professionals); be reluctant to name their problem as 'anxiety' or 'depression', and fear further medicalisation of their situation with tablets.

Patients *may* recognise the psychological stress of chronic illness as a cause of how they are feeling emotionally, with diagnosis often being a life-changing event that forces people to face mortality and potential disability. Adapting to a LTC is a constant source of stress to some people, with resulting difficulties in understanding how to manage it and feelings of guilt when not following lifestyle restrictions. However, not uncommonly, a person may have multiple interacting reasons for feeling low, including social factors, rather than just ill health alone. Other life events such as bereavement or relationship breakdown, unemployment and family problems may be considered as causes by sufferers, but not 'justifiable' ones as they could, in the mind of the sufferer, potentially be resolved by some action on the part of the person themselves.

Loss of health and fear for his future are likely causes for Hanif's distress. His view of these matters should be explored. His story also raises an important question about whether, since retirement, he has been able to establish a role for himself either in his family or in his wider social network.

## Case-finding

Systematic case-finding or screening has been advocated as a method to increase detection and improve outcomes for depression associated with long-term conditions. *Case-finding* differs from screening in that only those with risk factors for the disease are targeted. For example the New Zealand Guidelines Group advocates targeted screening in primary care for high-risk patients, which includes those with chronic physical disease. The Canadian Task Force on Preventative Care and the US Preventive Services Task Force also encourage screening for depression, but only where there is *Collaborative Care* available as a treatment intervention if depression is detected.

Simple brief questions exist for both depression and anxiety in the form of the PHQ-2 and GAD-2 (see Box 6.2). The Patient Health Questionnaire-2 (or 'Whooley questions') has been recommended as a screening tool in the UK as it was thought that it needed little training and had few implementation difficulties.

Box 6.2 **Case-finding questions for anxiety and depression**

**PHQ-2 (the 'Whooley questions')**
Have you, in the past 2 weeks:
- Felt down, depressed or hopeless?
- Had little pleasure or interest in things?
An answer of 'yes' to either question should result in further assessment.

**GAD-2**
Over the past 2 weeks, how often have you been bothered by the following problems?
- Feeling nervous, anxious or on edge.
- Not being able to stop or control worrying.
*Scoring:*
Not at all, 0; several days, 1; more than half the days, 2; nearly every day, 3.
Scoring >2 should result in further assessment.

Further assessment should involve the further exploration of symptoms, including risk, supplemented by one of the longer standardised questionnaires such as PHQ-9 or HAD-D for depression or the GAD-7 or HAD-A for anxiety to assess severity (see Appendices 1, 2 and 6).

## Management

There are three elements to the management of people with depression associated with LTCs in primary care: supported self-management, linking to non-statutory support, and primary care-based psychological therapies or medication. The NICE guideline recommends using a stepped care approach to the above elements when managing people with depression (see Chapter 4). Primary care is the mainstay of management for people with depression associated with LTCs. GPs and practice nurses can offer support with both comorbidities and integrate the physical and mental health management.

Rehabilitation programmes for the LTC may be locally available – for example, pulmonary rehabilitation for people with COPD, cardiac rehabilitation for people following a heart attack – and these may contain a psychological component. Referral to specialist mental health services is indicated at step 4 of the stepped care model.

## Self-management

Self-management is defined by the UK Department of Health as 'the care taken by individuals towards their own health and wellbeing' (Box 6.3). Depression can reduce motivation and capacity for self-management, and poor outcomes in people with comorbid depression and LTCs may reflect poor self-management. Patients are required to manage their LTC and may also be offered self-management approaches for their depression and/or anxiety. The increased burden of comorbidity should be considered when discussing self-care, which may not be appropriate for all. Regular contact will continue to be needed in primary care to monitor symptom level and progress and potential barriers to self-management.

Box 6.3 **Components of self-management**

- Healthy lifestyle – sleep hygiene; healthy diet; regular activity and exercise.
- Problem-solving strategies.
- Goal setting and planning behaviour change.
- Self-monitoring.
- Effective use of resources – including healthcare.
- Supportive social network.

Individual guided self-help is available in electronic forms for depression (e.g., MoodGym, Beat the Blues) or in self-help books. Self-management is not suitable for all patients. Hanif may appreciate some information regarding self-management; however, the GP might be unsure if Hanif is able to read this information (what is his level of literacy in English or in other languages?) or feel comfortable with using a computer for cCBT (computerised CBT).

## Linking to non-statutory support

Non-statutory forms of support include:

- Support groups for the LTC, such as stroke clubs, diabetes groups and local groups affiliated to the national organisations for LTCs (e.g., Psoriasis Association).
- National mental health charities, such as MIND, providing information on depression and non-NHS therapy.
- Local third-sector mental health organisations that provide long-term support to people with anxiety and depression including many that work specifically to help ethnic minority groups.
- National charities for LTCs, such as Diabetes UK and the British Heart Foundation, which provide information about the emotional consequences of LTCs and self-help materials.
- Religious organisations such as the church. Religiousness, although not spirituality, reduces the risk of depression associated with LTCs – perhaps due to a sense of group identity and values and support from other church members.

Knowing what's available and helpful depends upon local knowledge – what works as a support group in one place may be a fund-raising group in another. The local council often has details of organisations that offer support for particular LTCs (see Chapter 12).

## Psychological therapies and medication

Psychological interventions that are based upon the principles of cognitive-behavioural therapy (CBT) are recommended for depression associated with LTCs, and the Improving Access to Psychological Therapies (IAPT) policy initiative now includes treatment for those with chronic disease (see Chapter 10).

Structured group programmes that involve improving coping skills and self-management strategies for the LTC may improve outcomes for both depression and the LTC. Examples include the standardised cardiac rehabilitation programmes available in most localities, and programmes such as those offered to newly diagnosed diabetics, or pulmonary rehabilitation for those with COPD and anxiety.

All these produce short-term benefits for those who attend, but longer-term change is not usually maintained – possibly because they tend to over-emphasise education about the LTC at the expense of aspects of self-management or psychological aspects of the condition.

Antidepressant use is recommended for those with moderate to severe depression, or those with mild depression that is jeopardising the care of the LTC. Care needs to be taken with the choice of antidepressant as patients are likely to be on multiple drugs and interactions are possible. A full description of drug interactions can be found in the British National Formulary (see Chapter 11).

A patient with depression who has not responded to treatment, or with severe life-threatening depression, should be referred to secondary care mental health services for further assessment and treatment as with any depression. When assessing Hanif, the GP needs to assess the severity of his depression, the functional impact it is having on his LTC as well as his beliefs regarding the management options. If Hanif has difficulty accessing primary care management, has already tried this without success, has suicidal intention or the functional impact on his LTC is severe and life-threatening, then referral to secondary care is indicated.

*Liaison psychiatry* involves the delivery of mental health care in non-psychiatric settings. In the UK it has mainly meant working in general hospitals although there is increasing interest in developing sustainable primary care liaison services. The range is wide; well-developed services have multidisciplinary teams and offer consultation, advice about care, and outpatient follow-up in specialist clinics. For some specialist medical contexts such as transplant services or burns units, the service offers dedicated sessional time (hence the name) but more usually referral is open to all and treatment offered on a case-by-case basis. Limited resources mean that few services will accept self-referral or even GP referral, and access is arranged via referral from a treating hospital-based clinician.

Attempts to bridge the gap between primary and secondary care may include *Collaborative Care*. NICE recommends that collaborative care is organized for those with depression associated with LTCs that have not responded to initial management or patients with a high degree of functional impairment or impact upon their LTC (see Chapter 4).

## Barriers to effective care

Difficulties in managing depression include factors relating to the person, as well as professional and organisational factors.

*Patient factors* include denial of a problem, negative beliefs regarding medication for a mood problem, ambivalence to treatments such as psychotherapy, lack of resources to self-manage and concerns about stigma. Hanif may be wary of taking more medication or asking for help when he is already being perceived as being 'lazy' by his family.

*Practitioner factors* include beliefs contesting that depression is a clinical condition that needs medical intervention, particularly in deprived areas where the cause is viewed as social problems such as loneliness, being wary of opening a 'can of worms' during a time-limited consultation, viewing depression as a normal response to negative life events or justifiable in those with LTCs, and concerns regarding lack of skills to diagnose and manage depression.

*Organisational barriers* to take up of therapies such as CBT or structured group therapies for the LTC include practical barriers such as arranging transport and time to attend, or emotional ones including denial of a problem and potential stigma from attending. There is patchy availability for many services such as IAPT and structured group therapies for LTCs, and particularly for Collaborative Care within the UK, which makes access to such services difficult.

Relapse rates are high as depression associated with LTCs is a relapsing remitting problem. Social factors are significant, and perhaps play an even greater role in maintaining depression in this context. Hanif is likely to benefit from cardiac rehabilitation as this will help his fears regarding what he is able to do. Depending upon symptom levels he may also benefit from medication or psychotherapy for the depression. The challenge is to agree a course of action with him, and to find a response that acknowledges and treats his depression but does not over-medicalise it; it may take several appointments to negotiate such a position before an action plan can be jointly agreed. Longer term, Hanif needs to engage in a rewarding activity and develop a new social role. Further joint discussion with his family may be necessary to achieve this.

## Two neglected topics: the family and prevention

### Carers

Carers for those with LTCs, which typically means a partner, other family member or close friend, are also at higher risk of depression themselves. They often neglect their own health in their caring role. Clinicians in primary and secondary care have a role to identify those who are carers and enquire about coping, mood and mental wellbeing. Few services offer joint involvement of patient and carer in therapy unless the identified patient is a child or young person.

Families surrounding those with depression and LTCs also have beliefs that will impact on the sufferer. In this example, Hanif's wife accuses him of being lazy. An interview with her and with one of his daughters would help to clarify the role of family relationships in maintaining his problems. At this interview Hanif's wife should be asked about her own emotional state if possible.

### Prevention

We know little about how to reduce the number of people with LTCs who go on to develop mental health problems. Possible options include:

- *Public health* approaches towards mental health, such as promoting wellbeing in the workplace, debt advice and befriending interventions aimed at older people.
- *Early condition-specific support and advice* through, for example, specialist nurses or multidisciplinary teams.
- *Early acknowledgement of the risk* of mental health problems for patients suffering from LTCs can reduce the stigma associated with depression and encourage patients to disclose when they are struggling to cope.

## Summary

Depression and anxiety in patients with long-term conditions can be difficult to identify due to atypical symptoms and a reluctance on the part of the patient to disclose symptoms and the practitioner to explore further, so case-finding using standardised tools is recommended. Management consists of much more than just medication, but also ongoing support for the patient with an LTC from the primary care team, support for the carer, and additional services such as Collaborative Care intervention or referral to liaison psychiatry, to help overcome the barriers that currently prevent effective management.

## Further reading

Bower, P., Harkness, E., Macdonald, W., Coventry, P., Bundy, C. & Moss-Morris, R. (2012) Illness representations in patients with multimorbid long-term conditions: Qualitative study. *Psychology and Health* **27**: 1211–1226.

Improving Access to Psychological Therapies (IAPT) (2008) Long term conditions positive practice guide. Department of Health. Available at: http://www.iapt.nhs.uk/silo/files/longterm-conditions-positive-practice-guide.pdf (accessed 3 May 2014).

Knapp, P. & House, A. (2010) Depression after stroke. In: *Principles and Practice of Geriatric Psychiatry*. John Wiley & Sons, Ltd., pp. 515–517.

National Institute of Clinical Excellence (2009) Depression in adults with a chronic physical health problem: treatment and management. NICE.

Naylor, C., Parsonage, M., McDaid, D., Knapp, M., Fossey, M. & Galea, A. (2012) *Long-term Conditions and Mental Health. The Cost of Co-morbidities*. King's Fund and Centre for Mental Health.

## Resources

Beating the Blues: http://www.beatingtheblues.co.uk/

Royal College of Psychiatrists. Improving Physical and Mental Health: http://www.rcpsych.ac.uk/mentalhealthinfo/improvingphysicalandmh.aspx

SIGN guidelines. Non-pharmaceutical management of depression: http://www.sign.ac.uk/guidelines/fulltext/114/index.html

# CHAPTER 7

# Bereavement and Grief

*Linda Gask[1] and Carolyn Chew-Graham[2]*

[1] University of Manchester, Manchester, UK
[2] Research Institute, Primary Care and Health Sciences and National School for Primary Care Research, Keele University, Keele, UK

---

### OVERVIEW

- Grief is a normal human experience following loss – it is the emotional suffering one feels when something or someone is taken away.
- Abnormal, or 'complicated', grief is not uncommon, and is said to occur when the symptoms of grief are prolonged or more intense.
- 30% of people who are bereaved develop depression.
- GPs have a role in supporting people who are bereaved and grieving, and being alert to the development of depression.

---

Grief is a universal human experience following the loss of someone or something that is important to a person. It is sometimes confused with depression but may coexist with it. In discussing depression and anxiety, we need to clarify exactly what grief is and how and when it should be treated.

## Understanding bereavement, grief and mourning

Different terms are used, in everyday life as well as in the literature, to describe the experiences and tasks involved. We find the following definitions useful:

*Bereavement* is the experience of having lost someone close.

*Grief* is the reaction to bereavement. It is made up of a variety of thoughts, feelings and behaviours, which vary in pattern and intensity over time.

*Mourning* is the process by which we come to terms with loss and can re-engage with, and enjoy everyday life again. When it is successful, we find a place for the person we have lost in our life, and our memories. We will never forget them, but we can go on without them.

We never 'get over' the death of a person who meant a great deal to us, but we learn how to live with the reality of it.

## What happens when someone grieves?

Our relationships with people around us help to give our lives meaning, and are a source of support and pleasure.

Acute grief is extremely distressing and a time of intense and painful feelings. At first there may be a sense of disbelief and shock but this is followed by a range of different emotions (see Box 7.1). The acute period of grief can be difficult to distinguish from depression (see below).

---

Box 7.1 **Features of acute grief**

- Intense feelings of sadness and tearfulness.
- Yearning for the person who has died.
- Recurrent thoughts and memories of the deceased – sometimes accompanied by hearing the voice of the person. Memories may be triggered by everyday events or reminders.
- Loss of interest in everyday life.
- Difficulty sleeping and eating.
- Anxiety about the future.
- Anger about the loss (e.g., the dead person leaving them alone) or the behaviour of others (e.g., medical staff, members of family).
- Guilt – for example, feelings of having not done enough for the deceased, or not being with them when they died.

---

Over time, the intensity of the emotion begins to lessen. What is important to remember is that there is no universal rule about which 'stages' of grief the person will pass through and in what order. Five stages were famously described by Elisabeth Kübler-Ross: denial, anger, bargaining, depression and acceptance – but not everyone experiences these, and they were actually observed in people who were coming to terms with their own impending death (another form of loss), rather than the death of another. There is also no rule about how long it takes to pass through the acute stage of grief, certainly not the rule of '3 months' often cited in healthcare settings. The DSM-5 criteria allow for a diagnosis of depression just 2 weeks after a bereavement, and have been widely criticised as being over-simplistic and leading to the over-medicalising of a normal response to loss. Practitioners

---

*ABC of Anxiety and Depression*, First Edition. Edited by Linda Gask and Carolyn Chew-Graham.
© 2014 John Wiley & Sons, Ltd. Published 2014 by John Wiley & Sons, Ltd.

should appreciate key is the trajectory is towards lessening of the intensity of the grief as the weeks and months pass, and with time, a gradual moving towards re-engagement with what is going on in everyday life. Positive memories of the deceased can be recalled, and new memories can be incorporated into how we remember them.

Jess (see Box 7.2) is experiencing many of the features of acute grief following the death of her mother. She is able to gain some benefit from talking with her boyfriend about how she is feeling, but she also goes to see her GP.

---

**Box 7.2 Jess's story**

Jess's mother had a mastectomy for breast cancer 10 years ago. Since then she has been well, but when Jess telephones home at the weekend she senses that something is wrong. She has a close relationship with her Mum and picks up that she isn't her usual self. Eventually Susan breaks down in tears and tells Jess that she has been told that she has secondaries from her cancer. She had been trying to keep the return of her illness from Jess because she was doing exams, but now things are worse and she cannot keep it a secret any more.

In the next few months Jess isn't able to spend as much time with her mother as she would like while her mother undergoes more chemotherapy. Her mother doesn't want her to take time away from her course and they argue about it. Susan doesn't respond to the chemotherapy and her health deteriorates. Jess gets home just in time and is able to be with Susan when she dies. She is extremely distressed for the next few weeks, missing her mother terribly and feeling guilty that she didn't spend more time at home with her. She finds it very hard to keep up with her course and feels like she has lost interest in it. Her boyfriend, Oliver, tries to comfort her but Jess feels she cannot enjoy herself ever again now her Mum has gone.

---

It is important that Jess is supported in being able to mourn for her mother. Her GP reassures her and explains to her that the symptoms she is experiencing are normal and natural following bereavement. The GP listens to Jess talk about what happened to her mother and is alert to the things that might derail Jess's mourning such as dwelling too much on her negative feelings of guilt, gently challenging her views about whether she could realistically have done more for her mother. She checks that Jess is moving on in her grief by arranging to see her again a month later, and finds that Jess is beginning to take an interest in her studies again. She encourages Jess to talk about the good memories of her life with her mother and the positive ways in which her life can be remembered. The GP suggests that Jess might look up details of CRUSE on the internet, or seek further support from the university counselling service.

## When is grief 'abnormal'?

A small proportion of people who are bereaved, less than 10%, fail to grieve normally. People with 'complicated grief' show the features in Box 7.3.

---

**Box 7.3 Features of complicated grief**

- Sense of disbelief regarding the death.
- Anger and bitterness over the death.
- Recurrent pangs of painful emotions, with intense yearning and longing for the deceased.
- Preoccupation with thoughts of the loved one, often including distressing intrusive thoughts (and images) related to the death.
- Avoidance of situations and activities that serve as reminders of the painful loss.
- Feeling drawn to places associated with the dead person.
- Experiencing pain or other symptoms similar to those the person who died experienced.
- Hearing or seeing the person who died (this occurs normally in grief but doesn't usually persist).
- Suicidal thoughts and thoughts of wanting to join the person who has died.
- Creation of a 'shrine' to the person – often by leaving their belongings exactly as they were following their death.

---

Sometimes mourning does not begin and a bereaved person remains in a state of disbelief and shock regarding the death. On other occasions, the stage of acute grief may be short or the person may seem to function quite normally as mourning doesn't begin or seems to be suddenly curtailed. The bereaved person may, for example, be distracted by having to deal with family problems that arise following the death or in sorting out complicated legal matters relating to the death. The normal grieving process may thus be delayed and then triggered again (sometimes even years later) by a subsequent loss or by an event that powerfully brings back memories and reminds them of the loss. A further group of people may begin to grieve, but then remain very distressed, with this sometimes increasing in intensity with time; or the intensity may simply remain exactly as it was immediately after the death. Sometimes in such cases the personal belongings or room of the person who has died remain untouched, in waiting for their return. All of these patterns differ from 'normal' grief, where the intensity of the emotion experienced gradually lessens over time – even if this is over a period of years. Abnormal grief is more likely in the circumstances shown in Box 7.4.

---

**Box 7.4 A person is more likely to grieve abnormally if...**

- The death has been sudden or unexpected.
- The death was due to suicide.
- The person has been unable to view the body of the deceased person, or to be able to express appropriate grief at an early stage.
- There was an ambivalent or hostile relationship with the deceased person.
- There was a very dependent relationship with the deceased person.
- The person experienced difficult relationships early in life and loses a person with whom they found a deeply satisfying relationship.
- The loss involves a fully grown child.
- The person experienced a loss of their own parent as a child.
- The person has experienced multiple important losses sequentially.
- There is a lack of social support.

People with complicated grief have been found to be at increased risk for cancer, cardiac disease, hypertension, substance misuse and suicide.

Bridie, in Box 7.5, is experiencing an abnormal grief reaction. The intensity of her distress is increasing, and she is exhibiting several of the features in Box 7.3. With time, however, she also seems to be increasingly low in mood, and the GP needs to be alert to the development of depression and risk of self-harm.

---

### Box 7.5 **Bridie's story**

Maria receives a telephone call from her sister-in-law in Australia, informing her that her oldest brother, John, had a stroke and died in the night. John's wife is crying and obviously upset at the shock. Maria ends the call and sits alone, wondering how she will tell her mother, Bridie, who has never really got over the death of her son, Frank.

For the first few weeks Bridie is inconsolable. The family cannot not find the money to fly to Australia for the funeral. John's wife says she can pay, but Bridie isn't really well enough to go, so the family decide to all stay at home. Bridie starts to complain of pains in her chest and is taken into hospital. The doctor says she isn't having a heart attack and the pains are caused by 'nerves'. The family are all very worried about her and are not sure that they believe this.

Over the next 3 months Bridie becomes more and more withdrawn from the family and starts to sit on her own silently looking at pictures of John when he was a child. She gets very tearful when talking about him and says she keeps seeing images in her mind of him falling to the floor and hears him calling out for his mother. She feels guilty because she kept refusing to allow him to pay for her to visit because she didn't get on with his wife, and blames herself for not being able to go to his funeral, and for 'letting both of her sons down in life'. She isn't eating as well as she usually does and is losing weight. She doesn't want to go out to see her friends at the club and tells Jed that she wants just to join John and Frank in heaven.

---

## Bereavement and depression

Bereavement can trigger the onset or worsening of previous mental or physical health problems. About 30% of people who are bereaved go on to experience depression, and those with a personal or family history are most at risk. It is important not to mistake acute grief for major depression, but to monitor the progression of mourning in a person at increased risk for depression. If there is an increasing intensity and severity of low mood and clear presence of persistent symptoms of depression it may be necessary to *treat the depression*. This may also be necessary in prolonged abnormal grief if/when symptoms of depression begin to dominate the clinical picture, as is the case with Bridie. Bereaved people who are also experiencing depression may experience symptoms such as lack of energy, negatively biased thoughts and inhibition of positive emotions that interfere with their ability to move on in their grief and reconnect with life. There is no rigid time frame for this such as 'after three months'. Severe depression may become apparent well before this. In deciding whether to treat for depression it is necessary to continue to assess the progress of grieving and the emerging clinical picture.

## Treating complicated grief

This can be difficult; the bereaved person may feel that 'treatment' is not needed as they do not wish to stop thinking about the deceased and that any attempt at therapy is trying to separate them from the dead person in some way. It usually requires referral to specialist psychological therapy. However, some basic principles can be outlined:

- Help the person to both (a) talk about the past to try to come terms with their loss *and* (b) encourage and try to motivate them to re-engage with life by working with them using simple goal setting and behavioural activation. In the past, the usual approach to therapy with complicated grief was an approach called 'forced mourning', which focused on getting the person to talk much more about their loss. A newer approach called 'complicated grief treatment', which combines elements of motivational interviewing, cognitive-behavioural therapy techniques and interpersonal psychotherapy to address both (a) and (b) above, has been shown in a randomised trial to be more effective than interpersonal psychotherapy.
- Antidepressants will not be helpful for complicated grief in the absence of depression, but may be indicated if depressive symptoms are clearly present. A combined approach with both psychological therapy and antidepressant medication is most likely to be effective.

Bridie's GP listens to her talk about how she is feeling and realises that Bridie is not only grieving abnormally but is becoming more depressed and anxious. She is particularly concerned about Bridie's ideas of wanting to be with Jed and Frank. She gently explores whether Bridie has had any thoughts of wanting to take her own life. Bridie says she has thought about this, in order to join her sons in heaven, but her beliefs as a Roman Catholic prevent her from carrying this out as she thinks this would be sinful. Her doctor discusses with her the possibility of starting her on an antidepressant in order to help with the symptoms of depression. She also begins, at the same time as continuing to listen and empathise with Bridie's loss, to encourage her to set simple goals for re-engaging with everyday life, starting with simple tasks such as eating regular meals, and moving on to going out to see friends again. Bridie's mood improves slowly. She spends less time looking at photographs and more time again with her family, although she continues to have periods when she is very sad. Complicated grief takes a long time to resolve, and sometimes becomes chronic. It is important to try to help the bereaved person to engage again with everyday life whilst at the same time providing empathetic listening and support. Where depression is clearly present it should be treated.

## Summary

Bereavement can lead to a normal grief response. It is only when a person gets stuck in one step for a long period of time that the grieving can become unhealthy, destructive and even dangerous. Going through the grieving process is not the same for everyone, but everyone does have a common goal – acceptance of the loss and to keep moving forward. The process is different for every person and the support of a GP with time to listen and monitor can ensure that complicated grief or depression are identified early and appropriate treatment offered.

## Further reading

Shear, K., Frank, E., Houck, P.R. & Reynolds III, C.F. (2005) Treatment of complicated grief. *JAMA* **293**: 2601–2608.

## Resources

CRUSE. Support for people who are bereaved and their families: http://www.cruse.org.uk/

Royal College of Psychiatrists. Bereavement [leaflet for patients]: http://www.rcpsych.ac.uk/expertadvice/problems/bereavement/bereavement.aspx

# CHAPTER 8

# Anxiety, Depression and Ethnicity

*Waquas Waheed[1], Carolyn Chew-Graham[2] and Linda Gask[3]*

[1] National School for Primary Care Research, University of Manchester, Manchester, UK
[2] Research Institute, Primary Care and Health Sciences and National School for Primary Care Research, Keele University, Keele, UK
[3] University of Manchester, Manchester, UK

> ## OVERVIEW
>
> - People from ethnic minority groups have a comparatively higher prevalence of anxiety and depression.
> - Prevalences of long-term conditions such as diabetes, heart disease and arthritis are also greater in minority populations.
> - These comorbidities have significant implications on morbidity, mortality and quality of life of sufferers.
> - Cultural and linguistic barriers lead to poor recognition, help seeking and management of these conditions.
> - By recognising these barriers, developing strategies to improve patient navigation within the healthcare system, and developing innovative and culturally sensitive interventions, outcomes can be improved for these under-served groups.

This chapter considers the influence of ethnicity on the presentation and management of anxiety and depression, and explores the challenges clinicians face in responding to people of different ethnic groups with these common mental health problems, using the South Asian cultures as an exemplar group. Later we discuss the opportunities and innovations that need to be created within the health services to meet the culture-specific needs of minority groups.

## Anxiety and depression in people from ethnic minority groups

Anxiety and depression are the most common psychiatric illnesses amongst all ethnic groups. A high prevalence of depression has been reported amongst ethnic minorities living in developed countries. Research evidence for this high prevalence and associated risk factors mainly derives from people of South Asian origin residing in the UK and those of Spanish and Afro-Caribbean ancestry in the USA. This high prevalence of depression is also associated with reportedly higher episodes of self-harm and completed suicide amongst specific age groups amongst these ethnic minorities.

Among Afro-Caribbean people, rates of anxiety and depression appear to be lower in comparison with the general population, possibly because they seek help from alternative sources, such as herbalists or the church.

Depression in these groups is often reported along with additional symptoms of anxiety. As in any other ethnic group, it is observed that both conditions present with similar core symptoms but usually there are also culturally specific symptoms: south Asians in particular often describe 'sinking of the heart' or 'gas in the abdomen'.

Research shows that depression often follows a comparatively long-term chronic course among these ethnic groups. This may be attributed to complex intertwined psychosocial maintaining factors, poor recognition and lack of treatment-seeking behaviour leading to lack of restitution of symptoms.

## Culturally specific psychosocial risk factors

### Ethnic density

Geographical areas where ethnic minorities are densely populated have lower prevalences of depression whilst ethnic minority people living in low-density areas have reported a high prevalence of depression. This phenomenon may be due to the fact that people living in low-density areas feel isolated and there is more of a cultural gap between them and people living in their neighbourhoods. On the contrary, those who are living in high-density areas may find their neighbours more supportive, and there is a greater match between their cultural norms and those people living around them.

### Life events and difficulties

Research has demonstrated that life events and difficulties specific to ethnic minorities resident in the UK tend to persist over a longer period of time, are difficult to resolve, and are mainly related to interpersonal issues and physical health-related problems. The complexity of difficulties, and interplay between physical and mental health and social circumstances, is illustrated by the case of Robina in Box 8.1.

### Disclosure of symptoms

People from some ethnic minority groups may not recognise their distress as depression – for example, this has been shown in Black Caribbean women with postnatal depression – or do not even have the vocabulary to describe their feelings in terms of labels such as 'anxiety' or 'depression'.

*ABC of Anxiety and Depression*, First Edition. Edited by Linda Gask and Carolyn Chew-Graham.
© 2014 John Wiley & Sons, Ltd. Published 2014 by John Wiley & Sons, Ltd.

Box 8.1 **Case study: Robina**

Robina is 77 years old and has been living in the UK for the last 25 years. She only attended school for a few years in her native village. She lives in a city with a large immigrant population and speaks little English, always having relied on her husband, Hanif, or her son, Imran to interpret for her. Hanif is struggling with his health; he had a heart attack 3 years ago and seems preoccupied with his diabetes. He is always angry with her. Imran, her son, is always busy at work, and her daughter-in-law, Shabila, doesn't seem to be doing her duty to the family. As Robina cannot drive and has difficulty communicating in English, her movements outside her house are restricted. She feels very lonely even though the house is full. She is tired of being told what she can and can't eat, and wishes that her family would stop focusing on her diabetes. The practice nurse keeps ringing the house to ask her to go and have a 'diabetes check', but she doesn't feel she can go to the practice, even if her son takes her. When she was well, she could go back to Pakistan, and see the healer, she always felt better when she spent time in the sunshine.

People from some ethnic groups may be unwilling to disclose their problems to their GP. This may be because of stigma, but it has also been suggested that confidentiality is an issue, with some people fearing what they have disclosed to their GP might permeate into their community. Also it may be that GPs are less able to explore mood with people of some ethnic groups, and thus reluctant or unwilling to use labels of anxiety and depression. Robina (Box 8.1) illustrates the tendency to seek healthcare on return 'home', and GPs need to be aware that when patients return to the UK they may be taking alternative (or conventional) medicines.

## Health service-related factors

### Health services utilisation
Data from attendance of primary care reveals that people from ethnic minority groups, such as south Asians, tend to visit their GPs more frequently. However, these visits are more often for their physical health conditions and they consult their GP less frequently for, or are unable to disclose, psychological distress. People from other cultures may seek alternative care and support from within their community; fpr example, Chinese people may seek alternative care from Eastern healers, and south Asian people from imams.

### Pathways to care
South Asian depressed patients, particularly females, may consult non-health professionals because of low mood, and it may take longer for them to eventually seek help from the NHS. Self-referral to IAPT (Improving Access to Psychological Therapy) services has been shown to facilitate access for people from south Asian groups.

Services within the NHS are provided at different tiers and accessed via multiple and often complex pathways. Thus the barriers that can negatively affect the provision of services are encountered at different locations within the health service. The NICE guideline 'Common mental health disorders' outlines approaches that may be used to reduce the barriers and facilitate access to care for people from under-served groups.

## Clinical implications
It is important to consider the culturally specific psychosocial risk factors responsible for the higher prevalence of depression and anxiety in people from ethnic minority groups. It is also essential to note that this higher prevalence leads to poorer outcomes, not only for the mental health condition but for the associated physical conditions, which are also observed to be highly prevalent among ethnic groups, particularly diabetes and ischaemic heart conditions. Postnatal depression amongst South Asian groups has also been associated with poor physical health outcome and failure to thrive amongst children.

The UK Department of Health and the National Health Service (NHS) have recently emphasised the importance of meeting the needs of under-served groups. The document *Inside Outside* (see 'Further reading') calls for early recognition of symptoms, training of multidisciplinary staff to work with ethnic groups, and the requirement to tailor interventions to the specific needs of these groups to make them both more accessible and effective.

## Management of depression and anxiety

Primary care clinicians should take the opportunity to explore mood when a patient with any long-term condition consults, and can use the case-finding questions (see Chapter 4). The clinician needs to be aware that words such as 'anxiety' and 'depression' may not be familiar to patients of some ethnic groups, and so finding a common language is important. Thus for Robina (Boxes 8.1 and 8.2), an awareness of her social and family circumstances, and sources of information and understanding about 'mental health' are vital when she does attend the practice.

Box 8.2 **Case study: Robina (cont'd)**

Robina's daughter-in-law has been watching Urdu language TV channels and one day sees a discussion programme on mental health. She relates Robina's symptoms to depression. Shabila and Imran discuss this, but Imran worries that raising this with their GP would be stigmatising in the community. Shabila talks to Humah, who suggests that they should make an appointment with the GP and agrees to go and interpret.

The GP suggests that Robina could attend a local South Asian women's group at the library, and refers her to a local third-sector organisation that assigns an Urdu-speaking link worker with the aim of providing social support and introducing her to other groups in the area, including a diabetes education group at the local mosque.

The GP should also assess the severity of symptoms and discuss the use of antidepressants, if appropriate, as well as explore Robina's views of tablets. In this situation, the views of the family about tablets will be important. The GP should offer to review in a couple of weeks, and be alert to the pressure on the rest of the family – annotating the notes so that other clinicians in the practice are aware can be useful. It is likely that Robina will feel relieved that she has been able to share how she feels, and the family will be pleased that there is some help available, to relieve the burden on themselves.

Recognising the complexity and interplay of individual, family and cultural factors is vital for the GP to be able to support patients, and offer relevant advice, as Box 8.3 illustrates.

---

**Box 8.3 Case study: Nirma**

Nirma feels that she is not coping. Her husband hit her again last night and she feels she needs to talk to someone. She makes an appointment with a GP at the practice – one whom she has never met before. She is embarrassed to be attending and doesn't know whether her problems are something you should take to the doctor. The GP gives her time to talk about what is happening at home, and suggests that RELATE is something that she might find helpful (and that Naeem might also go with her). Nirma feels she needs to stop shouting at the children, and asks the GP if she can prescribe something to calm her down.

---

Giving a patient time to talk, although difficult in the 10 minute consultation, can allow the patient to tell their story and their expectations of attending. The GP should assess the severity of Nirma's symptoms using PHQ-9 (see Appendix 2) and GAD-7 (see Appendix 1) and whether there is any risk of self-harm. The GP should also assess whether there are any safeguarding issues, with full and frank discussion with Nirma if the GP feels that social services need to be involved. The GP might also discuss whether Nirma feels she should discuss her situation with the police. Additionally, the GP should be aware of any local women's groups and supported accommodation, as well as referral pathways for specific management of anxiety or depression.

## Models of care

The NICE guideline for common mental health disorders (CG 123) advocates the use of the stepped care pathway (see Chapter 3) for the management of people with depression or anxiety. The guideline also highlights other considerations that are important in managing patients from under-served groups (Box 8.4).

---

**Box 8.4 How to meet the needs of under-served groups**

**For the clinician**
Ensure competence in:
- culturally sensitive assessment;
- using different explanatory models;
- addressing cultural and ethnic differences when developing and implementing treatment plans;
- working with families from diverse ethnic and cultural backgrounds.

**For the service**
Assess local needs and respond by:
- assessment and intervention outside normal working hours;
- assessment and interventions in the person's home or other (non-traditional) settings;
- provision of crèche facilities, advocacy services, transport, bilingual therapists or independent translators; consideration of alternative technologies.

---

One particular model of care, developed for under-served groups, is the AMP model, which is described in detail in Chapter 12. This is particularly applicable to improving access to care for people from ethnic minority groups.

### Engaging the community

One of the main factors for delay in seeking care is lack of recognition in the community from the patients' and carers' perspectives. Initially people may not recognise the symptoms to be those of depression or anxiety; then they often seek alternative therapies (see Robina in Box 8.1), which may delay access to evidence-based healthcare. So, firstly there is a need to improve recognition, which can be achieved by educating people in the community using direct communication as well as working through electronic and print media. The focus of this educational intervention should not just be patients but the population in general, particularly groups like those suffering from long-term conditions, which are at increased risk of developing depression. The educational materials need to be in multiple languages incorporating idioms of distress.

### Working with primary care

In order to facilitate the passage of a patient through the service it is important for primary care staff to be sensitive to the needs of various ethnic groups. They need to participate in training in culturally sensitive interview skills. GPs also need to be aware of various voluntary sector organisations in the community (see Chapter 12) so that once the patient arrives in primary care they can be signposted to appropriate services (see Nirma in Box 8.3).

### Provision of culturally sensitive interventions

Historically provision of psychological therapies to non-English-speaking populations has been poor, particularly because of linguistic and conceptual issues. There is a need to culturally adapt these interventions to specifically address the problems in hard-to-reach ethnic groups, not only in the content but also the format, delivery, duration and most importantly the therapist's own training and expertise. In order to improve retention in therapy over a longer period of time it is important that provisions like venue selection, child care and transport are considered otherwise this may lead to poor engagement and attendance.

### Summary

A number of extra barriers exist for people with mental health problems from different ethnic groups. By recognising these barriers, developing strategies to improve patient navigation within the healthcare system, and developing innovative, and culturally sensitive interventions, outcomes can be improved for these under-served groups.

### Further reading

Department of Health (2003) *Inside Outside – Improving Mental Health Services for Black and Minority Ethnic Communities in England*. National Institute of Mental Health in England.

Department of Health (2005) Delivering race equality in mental health care. London: Department of Health.

Edge, D. & Rogers, A. (2005) Dealing with it: Black Caribbean women's response to adversity and psychological distress associated with pregnancy, childbirth, and early motherhood. *Social Science & Medicine* **61**: 15–25.

Gask, L., Aseem, S., Waquas, A. & Waheed, W. (2011) Isolation, feeling 'stuck' and loss of control: understanding persistence of depression in British Pakistani women. *Journal of Affective Disorders* **128**: 49–55.

Gask, L., Bower, P., Lamb, J. *et al.* (2012) Improving access to psychosocial interventions for common mental health problems in the United Kingdom: narrative review and development of a conceptual model for complex interventions. *BMC Health Services Research* **12**: 249.

Krause, I.B. (1989) Sinking heart: a Punjabi communication of distress. *Social Science and Medicine* **29**: 563–575.

Lawrence, V., Murray, J., Banerjee, S. *et al.* (2006) Concepts and causation of depression: a cross-cultural study of the beliefs of older adults. *Gerontologist* **46**: 23–32.

National Institute for Health and Clinical Excellence (2011) Common mental health disorders: Identification and pathways to care. NICE Clinical Guideline 123. National Collaborating Centre for Mental Health, London.

# CHAPTER 9

# Special Settings: The Criminal Justice System

*Richard Byng[1] and Judith Forrest[2]*

[1]Primary Care Group, Institute of Health Services Research, Plymouth University Peninsula School of Medicine and Dentistry, University of Plymouth, Plymouth, UK
[2]Derbyshire Healthcare NHS Foundation Trust, UK

## OVERVIEW

- Within prison settings, the prevalence of mental health problems approaches 90%, and of these, 40–50% have anxiety and/or depression; the remainder have a variety of substance misuse and personality disorders, with a small minority having severe mental illness.

- Demonstrating respect, care and concern; avoiding the label of 'mental health'; and taking a flexible, problem-solving approach can ensure therapeutic engagement.

- Management options for offenders in the community will be the same as for any other person, although it might be more problematic to persuade them either to take medication, or to attend psychological therapy sessions.

- Because of high levels of comorbidity and, particularly, the likelihood of substance misuse in this population, there is need for a wide range of interventions to be available across teams and sectors to enable continuity of care both in prison and beyond.

This case exemplifies many of the characteristics of those in contact with the criminal justice system who have mental health problems. They often come from socially excluded backgrounds, have ongoing social problems and have a range of symptoms across a number of diagnostic categories, in this case substance misuse as well as anxiety and depression. Patrick's anxiety includes both fight and flight responses, and he has been using street drugs as self-medication. He does not recognise himself as having a mental illness, or know where he might get help. His self-worth is very low and his trust in everyone, including the health service, has been minimal for many years. At 18, Patrick is probably too young for a diagnosis of personality disorder, which his troubled relationships might suggest, but later it may become a more obvious or defining problem. He would share this difficulty with many offenders.

This chapter will outline how, when dealing with individuals like Patrick, either in primary care or within a justice setting, there are particular issues that need to be considered in assessment, treatment and the design of services. Each of these will be taken in turn and background contextual issues are briefly outlined below.

### Case study: Patrick

Patrick had been arrested again – the police had caught him dealing drugs in the pub car park – he knew that his father would shout, his mother would cry and his grandparents wouldn't be told. This is what always happened. He was so angry that George never seemed to get caught, and this was his second arrest in a month. He thought that this time it might mean jail.

He also knew it was ridiculous. Yes, he had been using more and more cannabis to try and stay calm, but he didn't need to be so blatant as to do his dealing in the car park. Part of him realised that in a way he wanted to get caught as he didn't know any other way of asking for help. He knew that his mind 'wasn't right', but wouldn't have known how to explain it or express it. He didn't see himself as 'mental' and was certainly not as bad as the 'junkies and crack heads' he despised. His father was an alcoholic and he had often witnessed violence to his mother and taken a few beatings himself. As a teenager he had 'gone tough', trusting no one and building a group of lads around him who would do his bidding. But gradually, as he starting using street drugs, mainly amphetamines, diazepam and cannabis, there was a breakdown in previously good relationships with his grandmother, older brother and a couple of close friends. Now, walking through town, he felt like everybody saw him as a loser, and if they gave him a look or said anything out of turn, he could easily get into fights. Knowing this would end up with him in a police cell, he had stopped going into town and started keeping himself to himself, buying and selling enough cannabis to reduce his anxiety.

One day, by chance, when his doctor's surgery had asked him to come in to discuss his asthma, he met a GP who seemed 'alright' and when she asked him how he was feeling he found himself talking openly for the first time in many years. He described feeling useless, not being able to sleep and more recently losing weight and then answered questions about his poor appetite, interrupted sleep, low energy and palpitations. He was a bit surprised when the doctor said he had both anxiety and depression, and was very wary of admitting he was unwell and even more resistant to taking medication.

*ABC of Anxiety and Depression*, First Edition. Edited by Linda Gask and Carolyn Chew-Graham.
© 2014 John Wiley & Sons, Ltd. Published 2014 by John Wiley & Sons, Ltd.

## Background

Practitioners are often unaware that individuals have contact with the criminal justice system. Offenders may be divided into three groups: those with long prison sentences; short-stay prisoners, including those on remand, who have not been convicted and may be released at any time; and those with community sentences or contact with courts and police. In October 2013 the total prison population in England was over 84 000. While many of these individuals have long sentences, in the year ending March 2013, 57% of convictions were for sentences of 6 months or less, of whom 58.5% were likely to reoffend within 12 months of release. Twenty-six percent of offenders received a non-custodial sentence.

---

### Box 9.1 Mental health and social problems of offenders

Within prison settings, the prevalence of mental health problems approaches 90% and of these perhaps 40–50% have anxiety and/or depression; the remainder have a variety of substance misuse and personality disorders, with a small minority having severe mental illness. Those with anxiety and depression often also have symptoms diagnostic of one or more other 'disorder': post-traumatic stress disorder (PTSD); obsessive-compulsive disorder (OCD); antisocial, narcissistic or borderline personality disorder; and substance misuse, in particular alcohol, heroin and amphetamines. In women, self-harm as a part of borderline personality disorder is particularly common. Furthermore, many have symptoms but are sub-threshold making the total symptom load very high.

For those leaving prison, homelessness or unstable accommodation is common (37%), unemployment is found in the majority, and about 50% have children, though male offenders are rarely the responsible adult. These social problems are both their main concerns and motivators. For female offenders, care for their children is often a paramount concern and safeguarding issues are complex for practitioners. Emotional and physical trauma, as well as abandonment, are common antecedents of most mental health problems for those in prison, sometimes dominating their narrative, and likely to be key causes for the range of symptoms each individual experiences.

---

Care received varies by setting: general practice and primary care prison services are the mainstays of care for physical health and also for mental health care, mainly in the form of antidepressant prescriptions and fit-notes. Specialist mental health care is provided by in-reach teams in most penal institutions. Substance misuse treatment, which is funded mainly via the Home Office and often provided by a third-sector organisation rather than the NHS, is available to large numbers both in prison and those on community sentences. A small but growing number of prisons have their own Improving Access to Psychological Therapies (IAPT) services, and there is anecdotal evidence to suggest that most community IAPT services are ill equipped to deal with offenders such as Patrick, with comorbid substance misuse and symptoms of anxiety, depression and personality disorder.

## Assessment and formulation

While distrust and stigma might seem insurmountable problems to initial access, research with offenders in prison and evidence from services set up in selected areas show that in the right situation, offenders are often willing to engage with practitioners, services and treatment. There is compelling evidence to suggest that demonstrating respect, care and concern; reducing talk of mental health or diagnosis; and taking a flexible, problem-solving approach can ensure therapeutic engagement. Box-ticking and heavily protocol-based care with inflexible attitudes are less likely to be successful.

We suggest that formulations need to be based on a jointly agreed psychosocial assessment. An individual's background, including trauma, abandonment and other childhood and adolescent problems is important as is family history. An assessment of mental health symptoms is important to demonstrate whether individuals achieve the criteria for anxiety and depression, but in this group, screening for other problems such as substance and/or alcohol misuse, OCD, PTSD and personality disorder is crucial. We also find that some individuals may barely fulfil the criteria for anxiety and depression but have a range of other problems so that the total symptom load is very great. Many men express emotional turmoil as anger, so it is always key to discover whether this is masking other symptoms, such as underlying fear or feelings of inadequacy. It may be difficult to tease out whether offence-related violence is, at root, an expression of distress.

Comorbidity can manifest in a number of ways. Sometimes there are two clear diagnoses that need to be treated in conjunction but with separate interventions (e.g., depression and OCD). More commonly, diagnoses are interrelated in terms of symptoms, meaning and aetiology, and the formulation needs to reflect this. Classification of individuals primarily according to disorder in order to decide a treatment plan may not be the best strategy, and would not reflect collaborative effort between practitioner and client. Furthermore, diagnosis is likely to change over time. Anxiety and PTSD can often be revealed when substance use is reduced, or anxiety might return when depressive symptoms decrease and individuals become more active. In addition, individuals may feel more anxious in the community than in prison, or vice versa: both prison and community may be depressogenic and anxiogenic.

Developing a person-centred collaborative formulation should be based around an individual's personal goals, their strengths and preferred treatment options. Significant social problems such as unemployment, housing and relationship issues are likely to be much higher priority than admitting to having mental health difficulties. Rather than focusing on potentially stigmatising diagnoses it is important to explore the connection between the individual symptoms (thinking, emotions and behaviours) and specific social problems in order to determine whether and how treatment can help a client achieve goals. Assessment of an individual's strengths requires purposeful questioning. We are constantly surprised at how resourceful patients have been at maintaining their own mental health and any treatment needs to link with existing and potential self-care strategies. Figure 9.1 depicts the elements of a psychosocial formulation diagrammatically and emphasises the social.

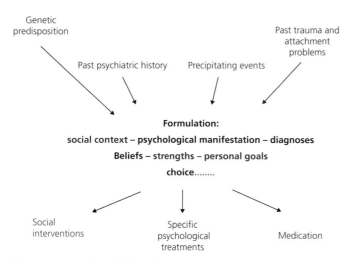

**Figure 9.1** A psychosocial formulation. Source: *Psychiatry in Primary Care.* Patricia R. Casey and Richard Byng. New York, NY: Cambridge University Press, 2011. Reproduced with permission of Cambridge University Press.

Lastly, the assessment should consider which services are engaged, or should be engaged, with the individual, who may already have trusting relationships with other practitioners. A joint formulation involving all appropriate services seems likely to have most therapeutic effect.

---

**Case study: Patrick (cont'd)**

Patrick's GP suggested that he might benefit from an antidepressant, and offered to refer him to the local IAPT service. He wasn't keen on either idea, and didn't collect the prescription. Then he got into another fight, and ended up on remand in the local prison.

On reception there he had a health screening with one of the nurses, who picked up on his anxiety and low mood, and extracted the information from him about what his GP had said. Patrick was discussed at the weekly multi-agency meeting, and it was agreed that he should be referred to the IAPT service in the prison; to the Drug and Alcohol Service for help with his substance use; and that he might be suitable for the 'managing emotions' group as a first step in coping with his personality issues.

The following week, Patrick met a CBT therapist who helped him feel that his worries and depression were entirely understandable and shared by many other people. When she explained how well medication and psychological therapy complemented each other, he agreed to try taking the citalopram as a 6-week experiment, as well as working one-to-one with the therapist.

At their next session, Patrick and Jane, his therapist, worked together to make a list of his problems and goals. He felt low about having let his family down, and anxious about what would happen to him. He couldn't sleep at night because of all the worries going round in his head, and he felt completely hopeless that things might somehow improve. Jane helped him learn how to control his breathing and relax his muscles, then visualise a place he loved and felt safe. Patrick couldn't see how any of this would help him, but agreed to practise every day 'as if' he believed it – the first of what would become weekly challenges.

His next challenge was to reduce his rumination and worry time. Together, he and Jane listed all the ways that he could keep busy,

like radio, TV, reading, drawing, phoning or writing letters to family, and cleaning his pad (cell). Over the week, he kept a tally of the number of times he did any of the things on his list, which helped raise his mood.

Patrick was surprised to find that with practice, the mindful breathing and relaxation actually helped, and his sleep gradually improved. In trying to comfort his family, he found relations with his Mum and Gran improved.

He began to set himself targets, like talking to one new person every day, to reduce his anxiety. This had the incidental benefit of helping occupy his time during association periods and he was soon playing pool, and going to the wing cv room, too. As his anxiety and low mood improved, Patrick's irritability reduced, and staff began to trust him to behave well, so he was asked to 'buddy up' with new prisoners on the wing – a real boost to his self-esteem.

---

## Management

Management options for offenders in the community will be the same as for any other person, although it might be more problematic to persuade them either to take medication or to attend psychological therapy sessions. Chaotic lifestyles do not lend themselves to regular commitments, and anecdotal evidence from the few wellbeing and therapy treatment programmes offered by probation services shows that client engagement is an ongoing challenge.

For offenders undergoing custodial sentences, there is a greater probability that they will attend for treatment (if only to get out of their cell for an hour, and to feel that someone is actively listening to and understanding them).

Medication prescribing needs to be approached thoughtfully, because prescription drugs may be used as currency in prison, bartered for tobacco and other commodities; or ingested in quantity in search of an illicit 'high'. Some people may attempt to overdose in order to have a trip out to hospital, whilst others will use it to self-harm. Prison nursing staff will carefully evaluate whether an individual should have 'IP' (in possession) medication. In the community suicide risk is particularly important – the most critical risk is the prescription of benzodiazepines or methadone, which in combination with alcohol and street-bought prescription drugs continues to contribute to suicide risk nationally.

All prisons will have a primary health team, usually including mental health trained nurses, but often the emphasis is on providing physical healthcare and prison mental health in-reach for severe mental illness. Some offer group work, for example for stress, anger or low mood (avoiding the stigma of 'mental health' labels).

There is little evidence to suggest that particular psychotherapeutic modalities are more effective than others in this group with such high levels of comorbidity. There is, however, a rationale for employing therapy that is able to address relationship issues (e.g., cognitive analytic therapy, mentalisation-based therapy). Anecdotal evidence suggests integrated services, where the interventions are shared in order to provide seamless care, are most successful. This is the case whether only one provider is involved at all levels, or in the extreme, where three different Trusts are commissioned to provide primary mental health, psychological therapies and in-reach, but agree to share work together. Still another organisation will provide substance misuse services.

The complex problems of the prison population and the limitations of the regime make working with this group particularly demanding. A common intervention offered by CBT for depression is behavioural activation, encouraging the individual to use activity to raise mood and encourage a sense of efficacy and wellbeing. If a prisoner is on basic regime, he may be locked up in his cell for 23 hours per day, and allowed only books (not encouraging for many with low levels of literacy) and a radio. This makes helping a client find purposeful activity a challenge. Similarly, recommendations to engage in outdoor physical pursuits will usually prove fruitless.

Therapists have to be imaginative in finding solutions – later in treatment, patients will often find their own ways round these constraints, but in the early stages, it may seem to them insurmountable.

Treatment for the many who experience symptoms of post-traumatic stress can present difficulties: a common option would be exposure to the feared stimulus, but this is seldom an option. Therapists may therefore use imaginal, narrative or other exposure approaches to enable the client to reduce the emotional content of their intrusions (flashbacks or nightmares). Similarly, phobic reactions that might be treated using the exposure-response prevention approach might test the therapist's ingenuity, although being given permission to go and disarrange a client's cell can be both satisfying and successful!

Finally, it is worth considering certification related to work. This involves difficult decisions that can have important lifelong effects. Few offenders receive psychological therapy and most obtain mental health care from GPs who as well as prescribing, are often asked for 'fit' notes. The combination of anxiety, depression and substance misuse, along with the old favourite 'nervous disability' are often used as diagnoses. The first note issued to a 24-year-old offender could be an important 2-week opportunity to have a break from the stress of work, but is more likely to be issued to individuals who are not in work, and is likely to transform into 3-monthly notes and then following external assessment to ongoing Employment Support Allowance (ESA). GPs need to really consider whether ongoing certification is in the best interest of the individual.

## Improving services

With such a complex patient population, there is a need for services to work together to provide integrated care across teams and disciplines. In prison, transitions between Steps 2 (mild to moderate anxiety and depression), 3 (symptoms not responsive to less intensive treatment, moderate to severe panic, OCD, etc.) and 4 (severe and enduring mental illness, or severe and complex anxiety/depression) must be straightforward and without delay. A variety of modalities is also important, so that CBT and person-centred counselling for depression are available alongside approaches to treating personality disorder (e.g., dialectical behaviour therapy (DBT) or schema therapy), and eye movement desensitisation and reprocessing (EMDR) for PTSD.

Another vital transition is for prisoners moving back into the community: research has shown that continuity of access is important, but equally so is continuity of information: there may be a

tendency for NHS and CJS systems to guard confidentiality, sometimes to the detriment of the individual being 'protected'. Flexible opening times and co-location with other services can increase the chances of engagement with services. Most important are the attitudes of the practitioners: a respectful, non-judging approach will do much to ensure the collaboration of service users, as will a determination to enable them to use their existing skills and strengths. All of these attributes are equally significant for those who are in the criminal justice system in the community.

Creating integration is complicated by having multiple commissioners for mental health care:
- Local Area teams for general practice care;
- National Commissioning Board, through specialised Local Area Teams for prison health;
- Clinical Commissioning Groups (CCGs) for community mental health care including IAPT services.

Substance misuse is often separately commissioned, with Home Office funding, and third sector organisations supporting wellbeing are commissioned by local authorities. Increasingly, though, prison mental health, primary care and substance misuse services are being jointly commissioned and tenders awarded to consortia of providers to work together.

New 'Liaison and Diversion' services are designed to ensure that individuals are assessed by police and in the courts so that mental health problems and learning difficulties are detected early. For those with severe problems, diversion from criminal justice to healthcare should be immediate, but for the majority, individuals will continue within the criminal justice setting. The liaison and diversion teams provide short-term input, including assessment, signposting and referral.

## Summary

Offenders are more likely to be socially excluded, to have experienced abuse or abandonment, to have multiple morbidities, than their peers resulting in a very high symptom burden. We have seen, however, that mental health care provision for those in the criminal justice system, whether on probation, on remand or in prison, is structurally deficient – both virtually absent and inappropriate. There is anecdotal evidence that recidivism rates are reduced where individuals have been offered treatment and support at vulnerable times. Research is needed to test different therapeutic modes and systems of care for individuals with anxiety and depression, coexisting disorders and social problems.

Anxiety and depression are experienced by many, in addition to symptoms of other conditions such as OCD, PTSD and/or personality disorder and substance misuse. Self-harm is a particular problem amongst women, adolescents and young men in the penal system. These conditions may be ameliorated or worsened by the individual's situation in prison or in the community.

The importance of person-centred formulation cannot be overestimated: working collaboratively with the client to take all psychosocial and environmental factors into account will enable a treatment plan based on the needs of the whole person rather than a particular diagnosis. This will increase the individual's commitment and engagement with the process.

Because of high levels of comorbidity and, particularly, the likelihood of substance misuse in this population, there is need for a wide range of interventions to be available across teams and sectors to enable continuity of care both in prison and beyond. Integration of the work of NHS, criminal justice and third sector providers will ensure that individuals will be given the best possible opportunity to progress successfully into the wider community.

This research was supported by the National Institute for Health Research (NIHR) Collaboration for Leadership in Applied Health Research and Care South West Peninsula at the Royal Devon and Exeter NHS Foundation Trust. The views expressed are those of the author(s) and not necessarily those of the NHS, the NIHR or the Department of Health.

## Further reading

Bradley, K. (2009) *The Bradley Report*. Department of Health, London.

Brooker, C., Ullmann, B. & Lockhart, G. (2008) *Out of Sight, Out of Mind: The State of Mental Healthcare in Prisons*. Policy Exchange, London.

Byng, R., Quinn, C., Sheaff, R. *et al.* (2012) *Final Report: Care for Offenders: Continuity of Access*. NIHR.

Department of Health (2009) *Improving Health, Supporting Justice*. Department of Health, London.

Department of Health (2013) *IAPT: Offenders Positive Practice Guide*. Department of Health, London.

Durcan, G. (2008) *From the Inside: Experiences of Prison Mental Healthcare*. Sainsbury Centre for Mental Health, London.

Edgar, K. & Rickford, D. (2009) Too little, too late: an independent review of unmet mental health needs in prison. Prison Reform Trust, London.

Her Majesty's Inspector of Prisons (2007) The mental health of prisoners: a thematic review of the care and support of prisoners with mental health needs. HMIP, London.

Howerton, A., Byng, R., Campbell, J., Hess, D., Owens, C. & Aitken, P. (2007) Understanding help seeking behaviour among offenders: qualitative interview study. *British Medical Journal* **334**: 303–306.

Prison Reform Trust (2013) Bromley Briefings Prison Factfile, Autumn, 2013. Prison Reform Trust, London.

Sainsbury Centre for Mental Health (2007) Policy paper 7: Getting the basics right: developing a primary care mental health service in prisons. SCMH, London.

Sainsbury Centre for Mental Health (2008) On the outside: continuity of care for people leaving prison. SCMH, London.

Sainsbury Centre for Mental Health (2011) Briefing paper 39 (revised): Mental healthcare and the criminal justice system. SCMH, London.

# CHAPTER 10

# Brief Psychological Interventions for Anxiety and Depression

*Clare Baguley, Jody Comiskey and Chloe Preston*

Six Degrees Social Enterprise CIC, The Angel Centre, Salford, UK

## OVERVIEW

- There is a range of evidence-based brief psychological interventions that can be integrated into routine practice.

- Helping patients articulate their problems and identify the things they want to change is key to enhancing the effectiveness of brief psychological interventions.

- Brief psychological interventions that help patients focus on behaviours and ways of thinking are particularly suited to primary care.

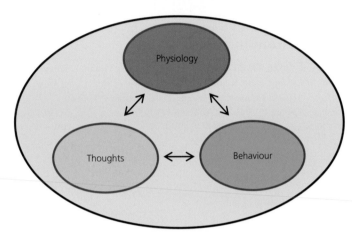

**Figure 10.1** The ABC cycle.

## Introduction

This chapter outlines key evidence-based brief psychological interventions, and explains how they can provide practical ways of helping patients develop strategies for managing symptoms of anxiety and depression. For a significant proportion of primary care patients, having timely access to brief, evidence-based psychological intervention will be sufficiently effective for them to progress, with a self-management plan, supported by scheduled review by the primary care practitioner. For those patients with apparently more complex or longstanding difficulties, brief interventions can provide a useful stepping stone to more in-depth and intensive psychotherapies.

## What are brief psychological interventions?

There is a range of options for brief psychological therapies, with 'pure' self-help drawing primarily on written materials, often referred to as 'bibliotherapy', and electronic or computerised resources, such as computerised cognitive-behavioral therapy (cCBT) packages that require minimal practitioner input.

Brief psychological intervention, often referred to as 'low intensity interventions', are based on the principle of helping the patient to develop skills in self-help approaches. As the evidence base continues to develop, the strongest models for brief 'low intensity' psychological interventions are for those based on cognitive-behavioural principles. These interventions focus on the 'here and now' of the patient's problems to gain an understanding of the triggers for, and maintenance of, the anxiety or depression in terms of thoughts, physiology and behaviours; this is sometimes referred to as the A

(autonomic), B (behavioural), C (cognitive) model of emotional disorder (Figure 10.1).

This understanding provides both the practitioner and patient with a shared understanding of the 'vicious cycles' of anxiety and depression, and offers a 'map' that can be used to guide decision-making about the best place to intervene to break the cycle, and the choice of intervention to achieve this. It can also be used subsequently to understand and manage stumbling blocks along the course of recovery.

Facing the challenge of balancing the principles of self-help whilst actively working to counter the inertia of depression or avoidance behaviour of anxiety, the practitioner works in a structured and active way alongside the patient to promote engagement and stimulate motivation. Using a combination of clinical skill and genuine 'empathic curiosity' the practitioner works to help the patient translate problems into achievable goals. To encourage self-efficacy between sessions, 'tasks' or 'homework' such as activity schedules or thought diaries are often used.

## What types of problems are suited to brief intervention?

Patients seen before their difficulties have become entrenched, or before significant secondary psychosocial damage has occurred, are best placed to respond to brief psychological interventions. In

*ABC of Anxiety and Depression*, First Edition. Edited by Linda Gask and Carolyn Chew-Graham.
© 2014 John Wiley & Sons, Ltd. Published 2014 by John Wiley & Sons, Ltd.

reality, most patients are unlikely to attend primary care for help with mood problems until they are significantly affecting their daily lives and function, such as their ability to work, or where physical symptoms, such as fatigue or palpitations due to anxiety, are causing them concern. Sometimes the reason for asking for help is initiated not by the patient but at the insistence of a family member or partner who can see the effects of the problems more clearly. Even then, because of stigma, patients may be reluctant to admit to being depressed or anxious and may not talk about their mood problems unless directly asked. Because of this it is very important that the practitioner has the skills to ask directly and sensitively about mood, is able to respond with an explanation that is supportive, and helps the patient develop an understanding based on a normalizing rationale that instils hope.

Whilst brief interventions are ideally suited to early-onset, time-limited difficulties, it is also possible to use the focus that brief interventions bring to complex or multiple problems. In particular the opportunity to gain early momentum around specific problems, by turning them into achievable goals, instils hope. This can prove to be a helpful measure in itself; by breaking the cycle of immediate distress and enabling the patient to draw upon pre-existing coping and problem-solving abilities, the brief interventions can provide the ground work for future psychotherapy for more pervasive difficulties. By using a stepped care approach (Chapter 3), low-intensity interventions can provide a basis on which to improve the 'here-and-now' situation, which will increase self-efficacy and in turn prepare the ground for psychological therapy to address the longer-standing issues if required .

Not all patients attending primary care will be obviously anxious or depressed. The case study concerning John describes a primary care patient, who is typically reluctant to ask for help with emotional distress but presents with somatic symptoms that they can more easily talk about. Importantly, unlike the scenario above, this patient does not have the observable indicators of vulnerability that would be more easily recognised. However, in reality, they are just as vulnerable, but more at risk of being overlooked.

---

**Case study: John**

John took voluntary redundancy 18 months ago. He lives alone in his own home, and was looking forward to having the opportunity to explore his interests. Two months after finishing work his widowed father had a stroke and John dedicated most of the next 6 months supporting his father in his recovery. His father has made a good recovery and regained his independence, but John now finds himself feeling depressed, without motivation and reluctant to leave his house. He is finding it difficult to sleep. He lies awake and worries. He has stopped seeing friends, and is reluctant to talk to anyone as he thinks he has no right to feel depressed and he is a failure.

---

John is interesting as, whilst there are clear environmental and life stage factors to account for his emotional state, it requires a degree of 'psychological mindedness' to manage this transitional process. John, although intellectually and practically able, does not necessarily have the skills to look after his mental health.

This is not uncommon, and the practitioner who encounters John in primary care will most likely be presented with the physical manifestation of his emotional distress, namely palpitations, insomnia and fatigue. This type of patient can appear to respond initially to reassurance about their health. However, as the underlying maintenance factors of inertia, avoidance behaviours and faulty thinking have not been examined the problem will be maintained and they will inevitably re-present or deteriorate further without support.

## Principles of working briefly with psychological interventions

---

Box 10.1 **Five principles determining care of a patient with emotional disorder or distress**

1 Ask directly about their emotional state and provide support where there is immediate distress.
2 Explore the problem in a structured way to gain an understanding of how the problem affects them as an individual.
3 Identify achievable goals and aim for early momentum.
4 Support self-efficacy by using the simplest evidence-based brief intervention first.
5 Proactively review progress at regular intervals and offer choice by discussing options.

---

There are five useful principles to bear in mind when formulating the care of a patient who presents with emotional disorder or distress (Box 10.1). It is worth noting that whilst each principle builds upon the previous, each may be therapeutic. Hence an enquiry that validates the patient's feelings and normalises their coping strategies, may be sufficient to provide the impetus for behaviours that create change, such as feeling confident to confide in a trusted friend. Or, providing a simple rationale for the way the patient feels, based on the interaction between how they feel, what they are thinking and how this is affecting their coping behaviours, may help them gain a hopeful perspective that has been impossible for them to achieve on their own. Let's look at each principle with examples.

### 1. Ask directly about emotional state and provide support for immediate distress

As illustrated in the case of John, not all patients will present with obvious outward distress, and empathic curiosity is required to elicit how they are feeling. A simple empathic and curious enquiry such as that in Box 10.2 provides a useful normalising bridge from discussion about physical health or social concerns to the impact on the patient's mental health and emotional wellbeing.

---

Box 10.2 **A useful normalising bridge**

*'It's not uncommon when people have been coping with the things you have just been describing they find themselves feeling down or anxious about things they would normally cope with, have you found yourself feeling like this recently?' ... 'What have you been doing to cope?' ... 'Is this helping?' ... 'Have you been able to speak to anyone about the way you have been feeling?'*

The key skills of empathic curiosity are:
- Active attention to verbal and non-verbal cues.
- Asking curious questions.
- Reflecting back concise summaries of what you have heard.
- Checking for accuracy and asking for feedback.

> **Box 10.3 Examples of empathic probing questions**
>
> 'It looks like just thinking about my question is upsetting you, is that right?'
> 'Can you tell me a bit more about this?'
> 'So you've been feeling down and worried for some time, but it's difficult to talk to anyone as you don't know how to explain what's happening, does that sound right?'
> 'Is there anything you would add or you think would be useful to tell me to help me understand?'

This stage is characterised by shared acknowledgement of the presence of emotional distress and the laying down of the foundations for further structured exploration of the problem (Box 10.3).

## 2. Explore the problem in a structured way to gain an understanding of how the problem affects them as an individual

A structured assessment of the patient's mental health is important to more fully understand the patient's problems from their perspective, help identify which are the key problems and decide what would be helpful to do next to gain momentum as soon as possible.

It is important that each patient is approached as an individual, and that the practitioner does not make assumptions based on their own knowledge and experiences. For example, John has experienced a number of stressors, each of which may be important in the development of his emotional distress. However, it may be difficult to disentangle the exact origin of the problem, and indeed the patient may not at this stage want, or be able to, discuss specific personal details. Eliciting the nature of the problem in the 'here and now' can be a useful starting point to map out the nature and severity of key symptoms.

Providing a summary and reflecting this back to the patient in the form of a 'problem statement' can have numerous benefits:
- It can help confirm with both patient and practitioner that their understanding of the problems/difficulties is accurate and clarifies misunderstandings.
- It gives a chance for the patient to reflect on the problem.
- It aides the therapeutic relationship as the patient feels listened to and heard.

Problem statements may be verbal, and the practitioner may encourage the patient to write the problem statement down (Box 10.4).

> **Box 10.4 John's problem statement**
>
> I have been feeling low and anxious for about the past six months since my father has recovered from a stroke. I am lethargic, have no motivation to do the things I used to enjoy, my sleep and appetite are poor and I have had palpitations when I am out of the house. I worry that I will never get back to my old self, and I think I am a failure. I avoid leaving the house; I've neglected repairs, and have stopped seeing friends.

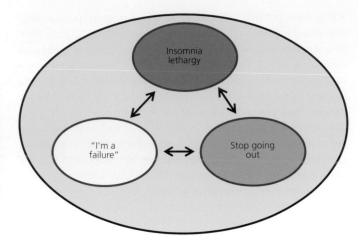

**Figure 10.2** John's ABC cycle.

A diagram using the ABC model may also be useful to draw out as an aid to providing a normalising understanding of the way that physical symptoms (e.g., insomnia, lethargy) interact with thoughts ('I'll never get back to my old self') and behaviour (avoidance) combine to create a vicious circle of inactivity, insomnia, avoidance and worry (Figure 10.2).

## 3. Identify achievable goals and aim for early momentum

A shared problem statement lays the foundations for a patient beginning to identify ways they want to move forward by identifying personalised goals. Goals are positively framed statements about observable things that the patient would like to achieve. They are an important part of the therapeutic process as they guide direction, break problems into small achievable steps and enable review of progress. Importantly goals should be generated by the patient, rather than the practitioner; this helps to give a sense of ownership and self-direction. Sometimes the very process of identifying goals is helpful in itself as it moves the patient from thinking about what they can't do, to what they would like to be able to do or have.

In order to be most helpful goals need to be 'SMART':
- Specific
- Measurable
- Achievable
- Realistic
- Time-framed

When asked the broad question 'How would you like things to be different?', John would most likely reply with the very broad statement: 'I just want to be my old self again'. Useful questions to help the patient turn broad statements into SMART prioritised goals are:
'How would you know when you were back to your old self?'
'What would that look like?'
'What would you be doing?'
'What might others notice?'
'What would be the best place to start?'
'Is that realistic? Could you break this into smaller steps?'
'How long would you like to give yourself to get to there? Is that achievable?'
'When would you like to review your progress with this goal?'

Examples of John's SMART goals following this questioning process might become:

'To be having something to eat at breakfast every morning by next Monday.'

'To be walking to the supermarket twice a week by the end of the month.'

'To email my friend Peter to arrange to see him by the end of the month.'

Once goals have been established they can be used to discuss the best place to start, which might be the easiest to try or which is the most urgent. This then informs the choice of intervention to be selected starting with the premise of trying the simplest things first.

## 4. Support self-efficacy by using the simplest evidence-based brief intervention first

Having developed an understanding of the nature of the ways in which the patient is affected there are a number of brief evidence-based interventions that focus on either the behavioural or cognitive (thinking) aspects of the symptoms.

### Behavioural activation

Behavioural activation (BA) targets the changes in behaviour that occur when a patient is stuck in a cycle of depression. This is often a good place to start with patients who have become withdrawn. The intervention focuses on gradually increasing activity by identifying neglected pleasurable, routine and necessary activities and scheduling their gradual reintroduction using a structured diary over a number of weeks. The key steps of BA are outlined in Box 10.5.

---

Box 10.5 **Quick guide to behavioural activation**

- Gather a *baseline* of current activity using a blank daily diary sheet.
- Draw up a list of '*Routine, Necessary and Pleasurable*' activities.
- Arrange the above list into a *hierarchy* making sure one from each is included.
- *Schedule* activities for the week ahead using the diary sheet.
- *Review* progress and discuss observations, e.g. what is helpful or unhelpful.

---

Behavioural activation is simple behavioural intervention that can be used with great effect to counter the inertia and withdrawal that goes hand in hand with the lethargy and lack of confidence associated with depression. With John, BA could incorporate his goals of eating more regularly, shopping and making contact with friends.

Some tips for using BA include:
- Work collaboratively with the patient.
- Write things down – use diary sheets.
- Break activity down into bite-sized achievable chunks – what would be the easiest thing to do first?
- Learn from observations – work out why things don't go to plan – then problem-solve obstacles.

### Graded exposure

Graded exposure tackles the key avoidance behaviour of anxiety. This differs from the withdrawal associated with the lethargy of depression as it is active avoidance associated with habitual pairing of a stimulus with the fear response, as in a simple phobia. This can be cognitively driven by an overestimation of the likelihood of the feared consequence occurring alongside an underestimation of having the resources to cope.

Graded exposure takes a structured approach to avoidance behaviour by encouraging the patient to gradually and systematically expose themselves to the feared object or situation in order to extinguish the autonomic fear response and help the patient reappraise their anxious predictions. In the case of John a programme of exposure may be useful for tackling his avoidance of leaving his house. By identifying an achievable behavioural goal the task can be broken down into small graded steps using the steps outlined in Box 10.6.

---

Box 10.6 **Quick guide to graded exposure**

- Make a list of all the things that are avoided – start with the easiest.
- Break down into *small achievable steps* and start gradually.
- Schedule exposure to *be repeated, prolonged and regular* – at least one hour per day until the anxiety response falls.
- Move to next step only when the anxiety response falls to less than one-half.

---

Some tips for using graded exposure are:
- Does the patient have someone who can help and encourage them with their exposure plan?
- Praise all success and encourage the patient to reward themselves.
- Encourage the patient to continue with the programme even on difficult days.
- Take a step down if the anxiety does not reduce and break down into smaller steps.

### Cognitive restructuring

Cognitive restructuring works on the thinking part of the depression cycle. Typically depression distorts thinking by selectively attending to the negative interpretations of situations or events, and minimising any information or observations that do not fit with this appraisal. The key features of negative thoughts are that they are automatic and they seem entirely believable at the time. Listed below are examples of typical negative thinking styles:
- all-or-nothing thinking;
- catastrophising;
- jumping to conclusions;
- mind reading;
- minimising or ignoring the positive.

Cognitive restructuring aims to help the patient identify negative thinking styles and thoughts; learn techniques to appraise the negative thoughts, consider alternative perspectives; and find ways of testing out or practising the alternative perspectives (Box 10.7).

The cognitive element of John's depression can be seen in his presentation; he catastrophises by thinking to himself that he will 'never get back get to his old self' and he negatively predicts that others will think he is weak for being depressed. By explaining to John the importance of thinking in the maintenance of his

**Box 10.7  Quick guide to cognitive restructuring**

- Ask the patient to keep a structured thought diary of automatic negative thoughts.
- Help the patient to spot typical thinking errors.
- Ask them to rate each thought according to how strongly they believe it.
- Discuss the evidence that supports and does not support the thought.
- Identify a more accurate appraisal based on the evidence and rate how strongly they believe it.
- Discuss how they could test out/strengthen this new appraisal – make a plan.

**Box 10.8  Quick guide to problem-solving**

- Identify the problem.
- Make a list of all possible solutions.
- Consider the pros and cons of all solutions.
- Decide on the best or most easily implementable solution to start with.
- Make a plan – 'What do you need to do? When will you do it? What help might you need?'
- Schedule a review of progress.

depression, and encouraging the use of a thought diary and using this to take a structured look at the evidence he is basing this upon, he can be supported to develop a more accurate appraisal of his situation. This might be something like 'I have had a very difficult time recently and it's not surprising I've been depressed, but with support there's no reason that I can't get back to feeling better.' With regard to his friends a more accurate appraisal might be 'My friends probably think I have had a lot to deal with. They will probably just be happy to hear from me.' This new alternative perspective can then be further explored by discussing ways of testing this out by planning to contact a friend and reviewing what actually happens and how this informs the new thought.

Some tips for cognitive restructuring are:

- *Ask about thoughts* – 'When you last felt down or anxious what was running through your mind?'
- Help the patient *highlight evidence that might be ignored* – 'What might be evidence that this was not true?'
- Use *behavioural experiments* to test out new thoughts – 'How could you find out more about this thought? What could you do?'
- *Reinforce by writing down* possible alternative thoughts.

## Problem-solving

A common impact of depression is that the ability to solve problems can be markedly impaired. Problem-solving is a very effective intervention to be used when patients are faced with problems that they feel unable to solve either as a consequence of their low mood or because they may have contributed to triggering the depression in the first place (Box 10.8). Sometimes situations or circumstances that require problem-solving are not apparent until they are exposed by behavioural exposure or cognitive restructuring. In the case of John he describes having neglected repairs on his house; further exploration of this reveals that the impact of this is that his roof is leaking and causing significant structural damage. Whilst this is work that is normally well within John's capabilities, depression has severely affected his concentration and confidence to think through and action a plan. This in turn makes him feel incompetent and embarrassed, leading to further avoidance and further deepening of his depression.

Some tips for problem-solving are:

- If there is more than one problem – *prioritise* the list – 'Which is the most important or the easiest to implement?'
- *List every possible solution*, no matter how unworkable they seem, before ruling anything out.
- If the patient finds it difficult to generate solutions ask 'What might you suggest to your best friend?'
- **Anticipate obstacles** – Ask what might get in the way of you doing this. And then how you could overcome this.

## 5. Proactively review progress at regular intervals and offer choice by discussing options

Typically the depressed patient will underestimate achievements and selectively attend to negative thoughts about themselves and their situation. It is important that the patient is helped to reflect upon their progress in a structured planned manner in order to recognise clinical improvement, understand what helps, and to notice when they not improving so timely action can be taken.

Some tips for reviewing progress are:

- Make a plan in advance (e.g., in 4 weeks' time).
- Use feedback from standardised questionnaires, such the PHQ-9 for depression (see Appendix 2)or GAD-7 for anxiety (see Appendix 1), and always specifically review risk.
- Review progress against the patient's SMART goals – what has been achieved? Are they still relevant?
- Praise all progress and efforts.
- Ask the patient what do they feel is helpful and unhelpful?
- Openly acknowledge and normalise things that are not improving – 'not everyone finds the same approach helps'. Discuss what else might be helpful – perhaps they could benefit from an approach that helps them explore the earlier origins of their distress, or one that looks at their relationships with others?

## Summary

Brief psychological interventions that focus on behavioural and cognitive symptoms of depression or anxiety are particularly helpful in primary care. Importantly the effectiveness of any psychological intervention is influenced by the quality of engagement, the degree of empathy and the extent of collaboration between the practitioner and patient. Goals are an important guide to monitoring change and intervention should take place within a care plan that incorporates scheduled review of change, symptom improvement and psychosocial functioning.

## Further reading

Bennett-Levy, J., Richards, D.A., Farrand, P. *et al.* (eds) (2012) *Oxford Guide to Low Intensity CBT Interventions*. Oxford University Press.

Myles, P. & Rushforth, D. (eds) (2007) *The Complete Guide to Primary Care Mental Health*. Constable Robinson, London.

Papworth, M., Marrinan, T., Martin, B., Keegan, D. & Chaddock, A. (2013) *Low Intensity Cognitive-Behaviour Therapy: A Practitioner's Guide*. Sage, London.

Richards, D. & Whyte, M. (2011) Reach Out. National Programme Student Materials to Support the Delivery of Training for Psychological Wellbeing Practitioners Delivering Low intensity Interventions, 3rd edn. Rethink – National Mental Health Development Unit.

# CHAPTER 11

# Anxiety and Depression: Drugs

*R. Hamish McAllister-Williams and Sarah Yates*

Institute of Neuroscience, Newcastle University, Newcastle upon Tyne, UK

---

**OVERVIEW**

- Evidence suggests that patients with moderate to severe depression, or anxiety not responding to simple psychological interventions, should be treated with antidepressant medication.
- Treatment with antidepressants works best if conducted in a systematic way.
- Consideration needs to be given to comorbid physical conditions, including pain, and substance misuse when prescribing antidepressants.

## When should the use of medication be considered to treat anxiety and depression?

Depression and anxiety are commonly comorbid and this can sometimes complicate thoughts around treatment. Fortunately the first-line pharmacological treatment of choice for both depression and most anxiety disorders are antidepressants, particularly selective serotonin reuptake inhibitors (SSRIs). There can be a perception that these 'psychological' disorders should be managed with 'psychological' treatments and that physical interventions are simply artificial crutches that can end up preventing the individual dealing with their 'difficulties'. However, there is clear evidence of biological abnormalities associated with depression and anxiety, and strong evidence for the use of antidepressants to treat these disorders. Nevertheless, it is important not to immediately jump to medication for any patient presenting with symptoms of depression and anxiety. The NICE guidelines for both depression and anxiety advocate a stepped approach to management, with antidepressants indicated at step 3, or when there is a previous history of depression. For patients with predominantly anxiety symptoms it is usually appropriate to at least try psychological and behavioural techniques (see Chapter 10) before resorting to medication. For patients presenting predominantly with depression the evidence suggests that if they have moderate to severe illnesses they will do better with medication than with psychological interventions and best of all with a combination of the two.

## Do antidepressants actually work?

In recent years there have been a number of high-profile publications and news reports questioning whether antidepressants have any clinically significant benefit in the treatment of patients with depression and anxiety. These have been criticised on many levels. A central issue is that in randomised controlled trials (RCTs) of antidepressants a large placebo effect is seen. As a result the difference in effect of the active drug often seems small in comparison. Conversely the effect of psychological interventions often appears large in RCTs. However, this is because such therapies are most usually compared against waiting list controls or 'treatment as usual'. In direct head-to-head comparisons in well-controlled studies, psychological interventions such as CBT are generally of similar efficacy to antidepressants in mild to moderate depression in working-age adults.

## How do antidepressants work?

The notion that depression is due simply to low levels of monoamines such as serotonin (5-HT) or noradrenaline, and that antidepressants work by increasing the brain levels of these neurotransmitters, is not tenable. The neurobiology underlying depression and the mechanism of antidepressants is more complex.

There is strong empirical evidence that stress can precipitate episodes of depression. However, not all individuals when stressed become depressed. The risk of developing a depressive episode appears to relate to the relative balance between resilience and vulnerability within an individual. One mechanism of resilience involves 5-HT neurotransmission within the brain. This system appears able to help prevent a negative cognitive bias. This type of negative cognitive bias is what is challenged in cognitive-behavioural therapy (CBT), since such bias can drive low mood and low mood drives negative cognitions causing a potential vicious circle. The 5-HT mechanism of resilience can be made vulnerable to dysfunction by a variety of factors including genetic and environmental influences. The latter include both early life adversity and current stress.

It is known that a range of different antidepressant drugs and electroconvulsive therapy (ECT) all have effects on 5-HT

---

*ABC of Anxiety and Depression*, First Edition. Edited by Linda Gask and Carolyn Chew-Graham.
© 2014 John Wiley & Sons, Ltd. Published 2014 by John Wiley & Sons, Ltd.

neurotransmission via different receptors or neuronal functions. The net effect appears to be common between treatments, that is, to enhance transmission in the specific 5-HT pathway that is involved with resilience and prevention of negative cognitive bias. This may help to explain the synergy seen in RCTs between antidepressants and CBT. The latter is challenging the negative cognitive bias in depression while the former is helping to support a more positive bias.

## How should antidepressants be used to treat depression and anxiety?

We have put together an algorithm that can be used when treating patients with depression and/or anxiety with antidepressants (Figure 11.1). It should be stressed that this is just one of many possible algorithms that could be produced and there is no hard and fast way that things must be done.

The starting point in treatment, as ever in medicine, is making a diagnosis. As described above, the decision to offer medication should be made for patients with moderate to severe illness. A patient's knowledge about antidepressants should be explored and any concerns addressed. It is important to review the patient and monitor the effects of treatment. In general, we are poor at measuring and assessing depression. One reason for this is a lack of consensus as to the best (and most practical) way of doing this. One possibility is to use the PHQ-9 (see Appendix 2): a score in excess of 10 would certainly be supportive of using medication. The decision to treat should, however, be made in a more clinically rounded way than simply on the basis of a score from a scale.

In terms of which antidepressant to use, there are a large number to choose from, but SSRIs are recommended first line. In our algorithm we suggest either citalopram or sertraline because these drugs have lower risks of drug interactions than fluoxetine or paroxetine and because citalopram is cheaper than escitalopram (Boxes 11.1 and 11.2).

---

**Box 11.1 Citalopram and escitalopram**

- Known as racemic citalopram, comprises two enantiomers (*R* and *S*), which are the mirror image of each other.
- It is thought that the clinical benefit seen with citalopram is due to the *S* enantiomer and that the *R* enantiomer inhibits this effect to some degree.
- Escitalopram (which only contains the *S* enantiomer) has significantly greater efficacy than citalopram. However, the difference in efficacy is only clinically relevant for patients with more severe depression or who have not responded to other antidepressants.

**Advantages**
- Well tolerated.
- Low risk of drug interaction.

**Disadvantages**
- Risk of dose-related QTc prolongation (but N.B. see text).

**Common side-effects**
- Nausea, vomiting, abdominal pain.
- Agitation, anxiety.
- Sexual dysfunction.
- Hyponatraemia.

---

**Box 11.2 Sertraline**

**Advantages**
- May give an improvement in energy, motivation and concentration.
- Low risk of drug interactions.

**Disadvantages**
- Often patients remain just on 50 ng, which may be subtherapeutic.

**Common side-effects**
- Nausea, vomiting, abdominal pain.
- Agitation, anxiety.
- Sexual dysfunction.
- Hyponatraemia.
- Insomnia.

---

Concerns have been expressed that SSRIs might increase the risk of suicide, particularly in adolescents and young adults. This could relate to the fact that lack of energy and poor motivation (which might lessen the chance of completed suicide) may respond faster than low mood following treatment. This is probably independent of class of antidepressant. If a patient has significant suicidal ideation it is important to review the patient after no more than a week.

For all patients it is worthwhile reviewing how the patient is tolerating the antidepressant at 2 weeks. The major issues to look for are whether they are experiencing problems with nausea, increased anxiety and sexual dysfunction. The first two tend to occur early in treatment and reduce rapidly over time. The latter, however, tends to be persistent. In the algorithm, there is a recommendation to increase the dose of sertraline from 50 mg/day to 100 mg/day after 2 weeks. This is on the basis that lower doses are better tolerated when first started. Although this principle has not been applied to citalopram, it can be considered in patients who have difficulty tolerating medication and in patients with high levels of anxiety. In these individuals increased anxiety in the first week or so of treatment can be problematic and therefore commencing the antidepressant at half dose and then increasing after 1–2 weeks can be helpful.

The main time point for review is then after 4–6 weeks. The evidence strongly demonstrates that if a patient has shown absolutely no response after 4 weeks, or minimal improvement after 6 weeks of treatment, they are extremely unlikely to respond to this antidepressant.

If the patient has shown a full response, the next step is to review risks of relapse (see Box 11.3). If there are no risks of relapse a patient should be treated for at least 6–12 months following full remission of symptoms.

---

**Case study: Maria's story**

Maria describes symptoms of a generalised anxiety disorder. She mentions that her brother killed himself, suggesting that there may be a genetic predisposition for her to suffer with depression. She is clearly struggling with her symptoms and mentions that she is feeling down with regards to her mood. If we assume she has a comorbid depressive and anxiety disorder possible treatments would include CBT and/or an SSRI such as sertraline.

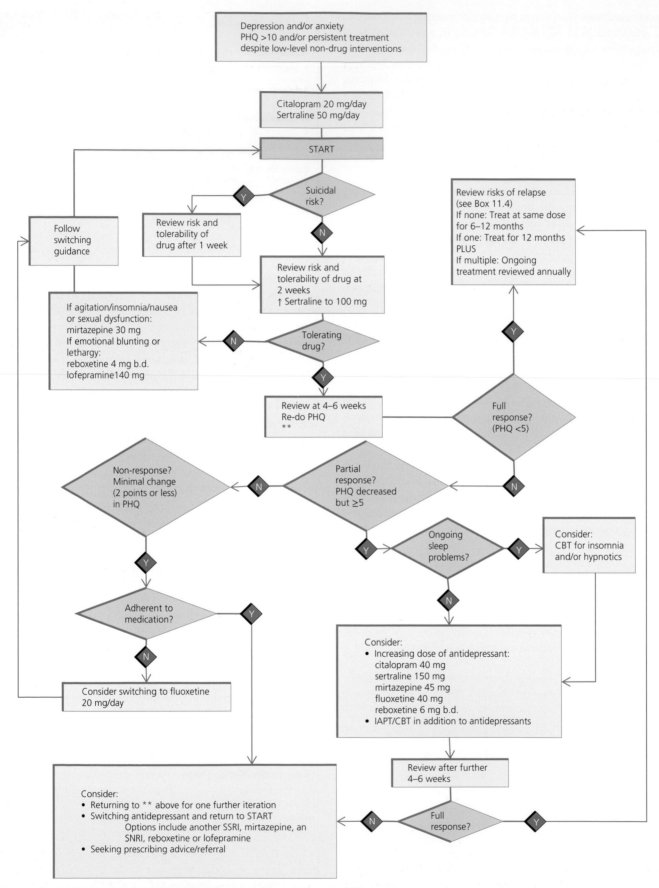

**Figure 11.1** Algorithm for treating patients with depression and/or anxiety with antidepressants.

Box 11.3 **Risk factors for relapse**

- Presence of residual symptoms – any increases the risk significantly.
- Number of previous episodes – high risk if 2–3+ previous episodes.
- Severity and duration – increased risk if severe or lasting more than 6 months.
- Degree of treatment resistance of the most recent episode.
N.B. Use clinical judgement.

If a patient has shown partial improvement it is particularly worthwhile looking to see whether there are ongoing sleep problems and addressing these either with psychological interventions specifically targeting insomnia or possibly using hypnotics such as zopiclone (7.5 mg) or trazodone (50–100 mg). Note that low-dose tricyclic antidepressants (TCAs) should not be used due to interactions between SSRIs and TCAs (see below). Alternatively or additionally consideration can be given for increasing the dose of the antidepressant (see Figure 11.1). It is then important to review again after a further 4–6 weeks to assess the effectiveness of this increased dose.

If a patient shows no response then the first question to ask is whether the patient is adhering to medication. If they are, the steps described above (for those patients with partial remission) can be considered. Alternatively it may be decided to switch antidepressant. This may also be considered for patients with partial adherence, for whom the antidepressant of choice is fluoxetine (Box 11.4) due to its long half-life (the active metabolite of fluoxetine has a half-life of 1 week). Alternatively if a patient is not tolerating a drug due to agitation, insomnia, nausea or sexual dysfunction, or you are looking for an alternative to an SSRI, mirtazapine can make a good choice (Box 11.5).

Box 11.4 **Fluoxetine**

**Advantage**
- Long half-life (reduces withdrawal reactions).

**Disadvantages**
- Long half-life (makes switching to another drug harder).
- Risk of drug interactions.

**Common side-effects**
- Nausea, vomiting, abdominal pain.
- Agitation, anxiety.
- Sexual dysfunction.
- Hyponatraemia.

Occasionally patients find it extremely difficult to tolerate SSRIs because they can lead to 'emotional blunting'. This refers to not only a reduction in the ability to feel sad emotions but also happy emotions. In such a case the use of a drug that selectively targets noradrenaline rather than 5-HT can be helpful, such as reboxetine (Box 11.6) or lofepramine (Box 11.7).

Box 11.5 **Mirtazapine**

- Different pharmacological action: noradrenergic and specific serotonergic antagonist (NaSSA).

**Advantages**
- Low risk of sexual side-effects.
- Sedative.

**Disadvantage**
- Sedative (N.B. sedation can be greater at LOWER doses).

**Common side-effects**
- Increased appetite, weight gain.
- Drowsiness.

Box 11.6 **Reboxetine**

- Noradrenaline reuptake inhibitor.

**Advantage**
- Lower burden of sexual dysfunction than that seen with SSRIs.

**Disadvantage**
- May not be as potent as SSRIs or SNRIs.

**Common side-effects**
- Insomnia.
- Sweating.
- Urinary hesitancy, prostatism.
- Constipation.
- Dry mouth.

Box 11.7 **Lofepramine**

- Tricyclic antidepressant that is primarily a noradrenaline reuptake inhibitor.

**Advantages**
- Better tolerated and safer in overdose that other TCAs.
- Lower burden of sexual dysfunction than that seen with SSRIs.

**Disadvantage**
- May not be as potent as SSRIs or SNRIs.

**Common side-effects**
- Insomnia.
- Sweating.
- Urinary hesitancy, prostatism.
- Constipation.
- Dry mouth.

If the issue leading to switching relates simply to non-response, then a number of options are possible, including trying a second SSRI or switching to a noradrenaline reuptake inhibitor such as lofepramine or reboxetine, a serotonin and noradrenaline reuptake inhibitor (SNRI) such as venlafaxine or duloxetine (Box 11.8), or a drug with a different mechanism of action such as mirtazapine.

Regarding how to switch antidepressants, we generally recommend abrupt switching from one to the other. This is possible when switching to or from an SSRI, a SNRI (e.g., venlafaxine and duloxetine), mirtazapine or reboxetine (i.e., most of the medications

**Box 11.8 SNRIs: venlafaxine and duloxetine**

- Serotonin and noradrenaline reuptake inhibitors (SNRIs).

**Advantages**

- Evidence for dose response curve – possibly due to increasing effect on noradrenaline uptake with higher doses (150/225 mg/day plus for venlafaxine; 60 mg/day plus for duloxetine).
- May be more potent than SSRIs (best evidence for venlafaxine) at higher doses and so useful for patients with treatment-refractory depression.
- Can be combined with mirtazapine for treatment-refractory depression.
- Effective for anxiety.
- Effective in reducing chronic pain.

**Disadvantages**

- Less well tolerated than SSRIs.
- Prone to lead to discontinuation symptoms (esp. venlafaxine).
- Can increase blood pressure (esp. venlafaxine).
- Duloxetine can interact with TCAs so don't combine and care when switching.

**Common side-effects**

- Nausea, vomiting, abdominal pain.
- Agitation, anxiety.
- Sexual dysfunction.
- Hyponatraemia.
- Insomnia.
- Sweating.
- Urinary hesitancy, prostatism.
- Constipation.
- Dry mouth.

listed in our algorithm and most commonly used in general practice). The only exception to this is if a patient is on high doses of antidepressants, in which case it may be advisable to reduce the dose for a week (or 4–5 weeks in the case of fluoxetine) before making the abrupt switch. Otherwise, with the exception of monoamine oxidase inhibitors, the only switch likely to be encountered that needs more care is from an SSRI to a TCA. In such a situation taper and stop the SSRI and wait 4–7 days (or 4–5 weeks if switching from fluoxetine) and then introduce the TCA. Further information can be found in the Maudsley Prescribing Guidelines.

## Prescribing with comorbid illnesses

### Cardiovascular comorbidity

In a patient with cardiac morbidity, prescribing can be complicated. The most important point is to avoid drugs that can lead to arrhythmias, particularly TCAs; these are also contraindicated in the immediate aftermath of a myocardial infarction (MI). There is evidence that SSRIs, in particular sertraline, can be effective in treating depression post-MI as well as reducing cardiac morbidity in such patients. This is for a number of reasons, including an inhibition of platelet aggregation.

Venlafaxine and duloxetine have a propensity to increase blood pressure. They can be used in patients with hypertension as long as this is well controlled. These drugs are not pro-arrhythmic and are safe in patients with cardiac disease.

There have been recent concerns raised regarding the risks of citalopram and escitalopram causing a dose-dependent increase in the correct QT (QTc) interval in the electrocardiograph (ECG). This potentially increases the risk of arrhythmias. As a result they are not recommended in patients with long QTc or at risk of arrhythmias. Recommended maximum doses are 40 mg and 20 mg for citalopram and escitalopram, respectively (20 mg and 10 mg in the elderly). However, it should be noted that in a large epidemiology study of several hundreds of thousands of patients, increasing doses of citalopram are actually associated with a decreased risk of ventricular arrhythmia and all-cause mortality. It is important to effectively treat depression for the cardiac health of a patient. If in any doubt do an ECG to check the actual QTc for the individual patient.

### Gastrointestinal complications

Selective serotonin reuptake inhibitors inhibit platelet aggregation and increase bleeding time. This is important in individuals who have a risk of GI bleeds, for example those on high-dose non-steroidal anti-inflammatory drugs (NSAIDs), and the elderly. In these patients, consider prescribing a gastroprotective drug. Venlafaxine and duloxetine have the same risks. If there is a major concern of bleeding, mirtazapine or reboxetine would be safer options or consider gastroprotection.

### Pain syndromes

Patients with depression are three times as likely to be suffering from painful syndromes as patients without depression. Conversely patients experiencing pain are more likely to be depressed than the general population. The presence of pain also makes it less likely a patient will respond to antidepressants. As a result higher doses and the use of SNRIs such as venlafaxine and duloxetine are often warranted.

Another issue that commonly occurs in patients presenting with both depression and significant pain (of any origin) is that they are started on an SSRI for depression and then have a small dose of a TCA such as amitriptyline added at night for pain. SSRIs, particularly fluoxetine and paroxetine, inhibit the metabolism of TCAs increasing their plasma levels. This can mean that patients in this situation end up with toxic levels of TCAs despite them being prescribed at low dose. In these situations it is better to either treat the patient with a dose of amitriptyline that would be therapeutic for depression (usually 100–150 mg or more) and stopping the SSRI, or switching both SSRI and TCA to venlafaxine or duloxetine, which also have efficacy in treating pain.

### Comorbid substance misuse

The management of depression in patients who are also misusing substances including alcohol or other illicit drugs is complex. In general it is best to be confident that the patient does have a depressive illness in addition to the substance misuse, for example, through observation that symptoms are present even when the patient is abstinent from alcohol or illicit drugs. In such circumstances antidepressants can be helpful, but in general it is difficult to achieve a good response unless the substance misuse is also addressed.

**Case study: Francis's story**

Francis appears to have an underlying social phobia. This has led to him using alcohol to improve his confidence in social situations. However, his alcohol misuse has progressed so that he appears to be dependent on alcohol and experiences withdrawal symptoms. This has resulted in his mood becoming low. Regarding medication in this circumstance it would be important for Francis initially to receive help regarding his alcohol dependence.

Recommendations suggest that antidepressants may improve mood but not necessarily decrease alcohol use in those who are depressed with harmful or dependent alcohol use. Generally mood will only improve in those with a significant depressive disorder, and use of antidepressants should be restricted to this population and then with caution and monitored.

## Pregnancy

It is important always to consider the possibility of pregnancy in any woman of child-bearing age when prescribing antidepressants. There are a number of concerns about the use of medication during pregnancy, which means the threshold for prescribing should be higher than in other clinical situations. Alternative options such as CBT or even ECT should be considered. However, if a patient is suffering from significant depression or anxiety it is important for this to be effectively treated. There is evidence that antenatal depression and anxiety has detrimental effects on the unborn child (see Chapter 5).

It is important to consider the patient's past history of response to treatment. If they have never been on an antidepressant, some drugs have more evidence to help guide decisions than others. This is not just related to the amount of time the drug has been in clinical practice. There are far more data relating to the use of SSRIs in pregnancy than there are relating to the use of TCAs. If a patient has previously responded well to a particular drug, particularly if this was only after failure to respond to others, there needs to be a good reason to switch to an alternative. There is no point in exposing a foetus to any risk if the drug doesn't work for that mother. Specialist advice might need to be sought.

## Prescribing to patients of different ages

The management of depression in adolescents is also complex. The evidence is that antidepressants may work but they may not be as effective as in adults. There is also the concern that there is a stronger association between the use of antidepressants and increased risk of suicide than in older individuals. The evidence base as to which antidepressant to use is also extremely limited. In general it is probably wise to seek specialist advice before using antidepressants in adolescents (see Chapter 2).

The same principles should be applied in the elderly as in younger working-age adults. However, there are a few extra things to consider. The first is that response to treatment can be somewhat slower in the elderly, and rather than making a decision to change an antidepressant at 6 weeks, it may be wise to wait and review after 8–10 weeks. A second is that the elderly or physically frail individuals may be more susceptible to side-effects. As a result it can be helpful to start with lower doses and increase these more gradually than one would do in more physically healthy individuals. It is important to judge the dose used against the response and tolerability of the individual patient. There is no inherent reason why an elderly patient cannot receive the same dose as a younger individual if they are physically fit. Finally, another consideration in the elderly is that these individuals may be on other medication and care needs to be taken with regards to drug interactions. For this reason citalopram and sertraline are better options than fluoxetine and paroxetine.

## Next step treatments

Having followed the algorithm shown in Figure 11.1, the majority of patients will show a response but a significant minority will not. There are a number of options than can be employed in such situations. The GP could consider switching the antidepressant for a second time. There are a number of antidepressants that have been shown to have a small but statistically significantly greater efficacy than others. These include venlafaxine, escitalopram, mirtazapine, amitriptyline and clomipramine. There are also theoretical reasons to think that duloxetine might also fall into this category. Note that this list includes two TCAs: amitriptyline and clomipramine. In general it is not recommended to use TCAs in primary care for the management of depression. This is due to their risks in overdose and adverse effect profile. The safest and best tolerated TCA is lofepramine, and this is a potential alternative to reboxetine in the algorithm. Otherwise amitriptyline and clomipramine are worthwhile options to consider for more treatment-refractory patients. Clomipramine is particularly useful for refractory anxiety disorders, especially obsessive-compulsive disorder or comorbid obsessional symptoms. In specialist mental health care, beyond switching antidepressants the next major alternative is augmenting or combining drugs. This will only be outlined here.

There is somewhat conflicting evidence to support various antidepressant combinations. The most commonly employed is the combination of mirtazapine with either an SSRI or an SNRI. These combinations tend to be well tolerated since mirtazapine actually reduces many of the side-effects seen with SSRIs or SNRIs. Traditionally one of the most common augmentation strategies is the addition of lithium, but this should only be initiated by a specialist. Lithium can be added to any of the regularly used antidepressants. An increasingly favoured augmentation strategy is the addition of an atypical antipsychotic to an SSRI to an SSNRI. In particular quetiapine now has a licence for this use in patients with a suboptimal response to antidepressant monotherapy. Again, such prescribing would be recommended by a specialist rather than being initiated by a GP. The GP, however, should monitor the patient for the metabolic complications of such atypical antipsychotics. While not licensed in Europe, there is also evidence to support the use of aripiprazole in such situations. Other augmentation strategies can be employed but they tend to be more used in highly specialised affective disorders centres. These include the use of triiodothyronine, L-tryptophan, modafinil and pramipexole. Electroconvulsive therapy (ECT) can be a highly effective treatment not only for patients with severe depression with psychomotor retardation and/or psychosis but also for patients with severe depression that has not responded well to medication. Further information regarding prescribing can be found in the British Association of Psychopharmacology guidelines.

## Further reading

Anderson, I.M., Ferrier, I.N., Baldwin, R.C. *et al.* (2008) Evidence-based guidelines for treating depressive disorders with antidepressants: A revision of the 2000 British Association for Psychopharmacology guidelines. *Journal of Psychopharmacology* **22**: 343–396.

Lingford-Hughes, A.R., Welch, S., Peters, L. *et al.* (2012) Evidence based guidelines for the pharmacological management of substance abuse, harmful use, addiction and comorbidity: recommendations from the British Association for Psychopharmacology. *Journal of Psychopharmacology* **26**: 899–952.

National Institute for Clinical Excellence (2009) Depression in adults: The treatment and management of depression in adults. NICE guideliine 90. NICE.

Taylor, T.P.C. & Kapur, S. (2012) *Maudsley Prescribing Guidelines in Psychiatry*, 11th edn. Wiley Blackwell.

Zivin, K., Pfeiffer, P.N., Bohnert, A.S. *et al.* (2013) Evaluation of the FDA warning against prescribing citalopram at doses exceeding 40mg. *American Journal of Psychiatry* **170**: 642–650.

# CHAPTER 12

# Psychosocial Interventions in the Community for Anxiety and Depression

*Linda Gask[1] and Carolyn Chew-Graham[2]*

[1] University of Manchester, Manchester, UK
[2] Research Institute, Primary Care and Health Sciences and National School for Primary Care Research, Keele University, Keele, UK

---

## OVERVIEW

- Anxiety and depression often have a large social component in causation and maintenance.
- People may not recognise their distress as 'anxiety' or 'depression', and may not be accepting of these labels.
- Some patients may have difficulty accessing traditional forms of mental health care.
- *Social prescribing* means referral to non-health-service resources.
- Primary care clinicians need to be aware of local 'third sector' services to direct patients to.
- New models of care may be required to deliver effective psychosocial interventions.

## The context

In England, the Social Exclusion Unit's report on mental health confirms that people from a number of groups find it particularly difficult to access help for anxiety and depression (see Chapter 4 on older people and Chapter 8 on ethnic minorities). In recognition of this, The Big Society was the flagship policy idea of the 2010 UK Conservative Party general election manifesto. The stated aim was to create a climate that empowers local people and communities, building a 'big society' that will take power away from politicians and give it to people, and supporting the development of local resources to support people in their community.

This chapter illustrates that collaboration between other organisations in the community outside healthcare (social care providers, public health, housing, local government and the 'third' or voluntary sector) is essential to ensure that people with anxiety and depression get access to appropriate help that meets their particular needs, many of which may have a large social component.

## Problems with accessing care for anxiety and depression

People who are experiencing anxiety and depression may not access care for a number of different reasons. Firstly, they may not recognise that they have a mental health problem, or do not wish to use the term 'anxiety' or 'depression'. Stigma remains a powerful problem in the community and militates against people recognising and seeking help for depression. Secondly, they may have difficulty in making sense of how the healthcare system operates (i.e., they lack *health literacy*), and understanding how it can help them. Thirdly, they may or may not actually seek help for symptoms, and fourthly their presenting symptoms and problems may or may not be accurately identified by a health professional (this is usually from a doctor or nurse in primary care). Finally, they may or may not be offered appropriate or acceptable treatment for their problems. Effective treatment for depression and anxiety is still lacking across the world according to the World Health Organization, and even where the evidence exists, such services or interventions may not be available for patients and their clinicians. Many people also have social difficulties, which are inextricably linked with their mental health problems.

## 'Social problems'

As we saw in Chapter 1, life events, chronic social stresses and lack of social support play a key part in the aetiology of anxiety and depression. This sometimes leads health professionals to assume that the mental health problems a person is experiencing and describing are simply a 'reaction' to social problems, are understandable, and not something that they (the health professional) can do anything to alleviate. This is because they do not think that the person can feel any better until their life situation improves (which may be wrong – they may still benefit from treatment that

---

*ABC of Anxiety and Depression*, First Edition. Edited by Linda Gask and Carolyn Chew-Graham.
© 2014 John Wiley & Sons, Ltd. Published 2014 by John Wiley & Sons, Ltd.

will help them to manage circumstances and stress more effectively and assist in their recovery). Additionally, they may think that there is nothing they can do to assist a person in actually managing their social problems – which is not entirely true. A key issue in medicine, and in particular in primary care, is the extent of wider social causes of health inequalities, which commonly accompany anxiety and depression and are a legitimate focus for health professionals. Many people with anxiety and depression have complex and sometimes enduring social needs (see Box 12.1). However, research has shown that GPs in the UK often have very limited knowledge of, and poor links with, resources in the community. GPs are most likely to refer people to counselling and specialist advice focusing on financial and housing problems, but much less likely to signpost people to community groups or to agencies that might specifically address other types of problem. Counselling in itself may be unhelpful if the problems that caused, or result from, the anxiety and depression are not in themselves addressed in a practical way.

Box 12.1  **Range of social problems**

- Difficulties with benefits
- Domestic violence
- Housing problems
- Unemployment
- Problems at work
- Loneliness/isolation
- Caring for others
- Drugs/alcohol
- Access to social services and other care
- Debt
- Weight problems
- Racial discrimination
- Asylum status
- Personal care
- Safety and fear of crime
- Bullying/intimidation/antisocial behaviour
- Children's behaviour
- Family problems
- Insurance/accident claims
- Other violence in the community.

## Social prescribing

*Social prescribing* may be beneficial to people with anxiety and depression. This means signposting people to non-health-service resources. At a time when budgets are being cut in social care provision across many countries, associated with high unemployment, GPs find themselves increasingly facing complex social problems associated with chronic physical and mental ill health. Medical and nursing professionals can play a role not only in providing information about resources (which requires up-to-date information locally available – preferably user friendly and easily available on the web) but also in supporting patients to make use of such resources (see below). Examples of such resources can be found in Boxes 12.2 and 12.3.

Box 12.2  **Examples of community resources**

Advocacy: welfare rights or mental health (provided by MIND in the UK)
Debt advice
Befriending services
'Arts on prescription'
Literacy classes
Support in getting back to work
Volunteering organisations

Box 12.3  **Arts on Prescription service for people with anxiety and depression**

**The 'Time Out' project at START in Salford, UK**
Start 'Time Out' Arts on Prescription service offers up to two sessions weekly, each lasting 2 hours with all materials and equipment provided. Professional artists are there to help as much as members need and will guide them through a series of activities, which could include: drawing and painting, pottery, gardening, photography and more. They can try a variety of activities and choose what they like best. Beginners are especially welcome.

The project is flexible and can last up to 6 months. Members can explore opportunities in volunteering, leisure interests, employment and education. Or, having enjoyed their 6 months of art sessions they may then decide to join the member-led art group.

A mental health worker carries out the initial assessment, and is available for one-to-one counselling and support when needed. She also runs workshops to promote mental wellbeing such as relaxation sessions.

Additional outreach art sessions are also organised in local primary care settings, which have also welcomed exhibitions of members' work.

Research into the Arts on Prescription initiative described in Box 12.3 revealed it provided 'added value' over and above being in receipt of psychological therapy alone. People attending perceived themselves as 'returning to normality' through enjoying life again, returning to previous activities, setting goals and stopping dwelling on the past, which for many had been a negative experience of more 'talking' approaches to therapy.

Finding evidence of 'hard' outcomes, in terms of cost-effectiveness, for social prescribing is difficult, although it has been shown to have an impact on anxiety, general health and quality of life in a large randomised controlled trial conducted some years ago in the UK by Grant and colleagues. Such interventions may be more acceptable to some groups – e.g., older people and people from British Minority Ethnic (BME) communities. There is also evidence that 'befriending' interventions are effective in reducing depression in older people, possibly by reducing loneliness that many older people experience.

## Improving access

We think that improving access to care in the community for anxiety and depression requires a multifaceted approach (Figure 12.1) with three linked components: community engagement; addressing the

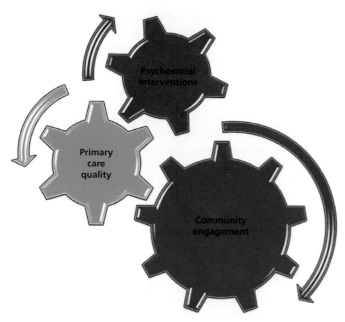

**Figure 12.1** Multifaceted model to improve access to mental health care.

quality of primary care; and providing psychosocial interventions that are tailored to the needs of people with complex reasons why they may have difficulty in accessing care.

- *Community engagement*: means working in partnership with existing third-sector agencies, such a local black and ethnic minority organisations, services for older people, teenagers, asylum seekers and homeless people. Many of the people working in these organisations have a great deal of experience in trying to help people with anxiety and depression to access care. They may, however, have difficulty making links with traditional health providers such as primary care. They also may sometimes lack resources and expertise to be able to provide evidence-based and well-supervised psychological interventions, and again would benefit from closer links with mental health care providers. Third-sector workers are able to help identify areas of unmet need and, in our experience, are keen to improve their links with primary care to enable this.
- *Addressing the quality of primary care*: needs to consider the experiences of people with anxiety and depression from the moment they approach the medical practice to register as a patient through contacting the reception for an appointment and visiting the doctor or nurse. What are the particular barriers to access in the practice? How does the receptionist manage a person who is in crisis, irritable and very anxious, at the front counter, and who does not seem to understand English? Are self-help materials for patients available in a range of languages? What about people who are illiterate? Is the practice team culturally competent? How much does the team know about the broad range of services available in the community (see 'Social prescribing' above).
- *Providing tailored psychosocial interventions*: there is evidence for the effectiveness of tailored psychosocial interventions for some groups, particularly older people and ethnic minorities (see Chapters 4 and 8). Tailoring needs to be based on an understanding of the factors that influence people's response to an

intervention and usually involves addressing social aspects of the format, content and delivery of, for example, a group without interfering with key aspects of the psychological content that are necessary for the effectiveness of the intervention. The term 'mental health' may, for example, be unacceptable to some groups. In an intervention for people from the Jewish community in Manchester, the groups that we set up for people to support self-help for anxiety and depression were called 'personal development' groups – which was a far more acceptable term. Sometimes 'wellbeing' is used, but we have found that people still equate this to 'mental health', and do not find it an acceptable term. Community organisations should be both involved in designing and be partners in providing these interventions.

In Box 12.4 we can see how Anthony, Bridie's husband, is engaged in accessing help for his anxiety and depression through a combination of effective collaboration between the third sector and healthcare (local advertising of an outreach resource in the community in a healthcare waiting room, encouragement from a healthcare practitioner who recognises Anthony's problem and knows about what is available in the community) and the availability of a tailored resource in the community (a service that will, if necessary visit at home, which for some older people is essential, though not for Anthony, and that runs groups that are not stigmatising – 'craft and

---

**Box 12.4 Case study in working together with the community: Anthony (senior)**

Anthony, Bridie's husband, has never been very good at telling people how he feels. He has managed to cope with all of the problems within his family and always been strong for everyone. However, since the death of his son his wife has been much lower in mood. At one time they used to enjoy doing things together, going out and seeing friends. He also had several hobbies. Woodworking and fishing were his favourites. Now he rarely goes out.

Maria has seen an advertisement on the noticeboard at the GP's clinic for a service offering help for older people who are feeling unhappy or stressed. She thinks it would be good for her father, to give him some support, but he isn't at all keen to go, saying he isn't 'mental'. However, when he next sees the practice nurse for a check up on his blood pressure she mentions it too. He says he will think about it, and she asks if it is OK for the worker from the service to contact him.

Anthony eventually agrees to see Brenda, the Psychological Well-Being Practitioner, who is working with a third-sector organisation in the community. She would have been willing to see him at home, but he insists they meet at the doctor's as he doesn't want anyone in the street to see her visiting.

Brenda asks Anthony to complete some questionnaires. His PHQ-9 score is 17 and his GAD-7 is 12. To his surprise, Anthony is able to talk easily with Brenda, and he shares how much he has missed his friends and his hobbies since he retired from work and has to spend more time taking care of Bridie. They meet three or four times, and Brenda is able to work with him using behavioural activation to increase his activity. She manages to persuade him to join a 'craft and chat' group at the local Age Concern centre.

Six months later, Anthony is volunteering at the Centre, and helping to run the fishing group. He is feeling much better. His PHQ-9 score is now 8 and his GAD-7 score is 10.

chat'). Elements of the AMP (Improving Access to Mental Health in Primary Care) model (quality of primary care, tailored psychosocial interventions) can be identified here. The important groundwork involved in commissioning the elements of the intervention and ensuring that key stakeholders (including primary care) were involved in designing and setting up the pathways that enable this to work constitutes the 'community engagement'.

## Summary

Primary care clinicians play an important role in the diagnosis and support of people with anxiety and depression, but need to harness the resources of their local community, signposting people to appropriate and acceptable services, tailored to meet the needs of specific patient groups.

## Further reading

Brandling, J. & House, W. (2009) Social prescribing in general practice: adding meaning to medicine. *British Journal of General Practice* **59**: 454.

Gask, L., Bower, P., Lamb, J. *et al.* (2012) Improving access to psychosocial interventions for common mental health problems in the United Kingdom: narrative review and development of a conceptual model for complex interventions. *BMC Health Services Research* **12**: 249.

Grant, C., Goodenough, T., Harvey, I. & Hine, C. (2000) A randomised controlled trial and economic evaluation of a referrals facilitator between primary care and the voluntary sector. *British Medical Journal* **320**: 419–423.

Makin, S. & Gask, L. (2012) 'Getting back to normal': the added value of an art-based programme in promoting 'recovery' for common but chronic mental health problems. *Chronic Illness* **8**: 64–75.

Popay, J., Kowarzik, U., Mallinson, S., Mackian, S. & Barker, J. (2007) Social problems, primary care and pathways to help and support: addressing health inequalities at the individual level. Part I: the GP perspective. *Journal of Epidemiology and Community Health* **61**: 966–971.

Social Exclusion Unit (2004) Mental health and social exclusion. London: Office of the Deputy Prime Minister.

## Resource

Information about the AMP project (Improving Access to Mental Health in Primary Care) can be found at www.amproject.org.uk

# CHAPTER 13

# Looking After Ourselves

*Ceri Dornan[1] and Louise Ivinson[2]*

[1]Honorary Secretary, UK Balint Society; email: contact@balint.co.uk
[2]Scottish Association of Psychoanalytical Psychotherapists/British Psychoanalytic Council, 19–23 Wedmore Street, London, UK

---

## OVERVIEW

- Health professionals face complex emotional demands in their work.
- Many clinicians find it very hard to ask for the help they need.
- How can health professionals become more resilient?
- How can clinicians help each other?

---

The previous chapters illustrate how intertwined physical and mental health, economic and social circumstances, and personal lives can be. Difficult economic circumstances have had a particular impact on the population's mental health. These factors contribute to a complex working environment for healthcare professionals and a heavy emotional load, combined with the impact of the many changes required as a result of external policies. The chapter is written with GPs in mind, but the same principles apply to other health care professionals.

Being a doctor is not always good for your health. The statistics for burnout, depression, substance abuse and suicide indicate that, despite the socioeconomic advantages of the profession, doctors are at risk. Doctor support services report that the age of people contacting them has decreased in recent years. Doctors are late to seek help and it may only be when there are concerns about fitness to practise that problems come to light. There does seem to be a need to encourage clinicians to be more aware of what is happening to them, and much sooner. Many organisations are concerned about this topic, as illustrated by the resource list at the end of this chapter. There are succinct summaries of the reasons for concern, so rather than repeat these, we would like to focus on issues of vulnerability and resilience, and offer you a space to think about yourself as an individual, in relation to your work. We bring the perspectives of a recently retired GP with an interest in mental health, and a psychiatrist, now practising as a psychoanalytic psychotherapist. We have worked together as co-leaders of a GP Balint group. What follows is the result of several conversations in which we have tried to answer these questions:

- Why do some people seem to be more vulnerable to the impact of their work pressures than others?
- Why is it so difficult for doctors to ask for help?
- Can resilience be developed, or are we just the way we are?

## Why do some people seem to be more vulnerable to the impact of their work pressures than others?

Maybe we should start by thinking about what draws people to become health professionals, despite it being an arena of illness, trauma and death. There will be a variety of conscious reasons, such as parents' profession, early experience of health settings either personally or through family illness, through to interest in science and people, and a desire to make a difference to others. A psychoanalytic perspective suggests that there are less conscious reasons, which may contribute to vulnerability or resilience. It is worth stating here that what follows is simplified to make a point, and that there are many factors governing how we 'turn out'.

The development of our internal world, or what is in our conscious and unconscious mind, can be thought of as happening in the presence of a maternal, nurturing influence and a more intellectual, world-orientated, critical paternal one. These do not have to be actual parents, or indeed specific male or female figures. For a healthy, balanced internal world, infants need to experience responsive caring such that they are not left feeling inadequately 'nourished'. They also need to be kept 'safe enough', physically and emotionally, so that they can develop the confidence to pursue developmentally appropriate challenges, accepting that frustrations and mistakes will occur. In time they will be able to reflect upon, own and understand their limitations without undue recrimination of themselves or others. Many of us can hear that over-critical voice inside us, or 'self-talk' as it is sometimes described, and occasionally remember where that voice originated from. 'You must try harder', 'I expected better of you', 'Failure is not an option', as opposed to 'You can't get it right every time', 'You tried your best', 'OK, that was a silly mistake, but you will know better next time' or 'Have another try'.

What can happen if we do not feel adequately 'nourished'? We may then seek nourishment from others, for example in close relationships. Or, we may be drawn into situations of caring for others. By looking after others, we are actually looking after a part of ourselves. This might work, but there are risks. One is that there is confusion between the needs of the other person and our own needs. Another is that we desire gratitude and evidence of success in order

---

*ABC of Anxiety and Depression*, First Edition. Edited by Linda Gask and Carolyn Chew-Graham.
© 2014 John Wiley & Sons, Ltd. Published 2014 by John Wiley & Sons, Ltd.

to make us feel good, or 'nourished'. It is easy to see how in the real world of healthcare practice, where many problems do not have solutions that we can influence, or the other person will not or cannot offer us gratitude, we are going to be disappointed.

Let us imagine two fictitious doctors with contrasting emotional worlds. The first GP is quite emotionally articulate, in contact with their feelings but at risk of these becoming 'too much' and may be perceived by others as over-involved with 'needy' patients. This doctor grapples with excessive guilt, an overdeveloped sense of responsibility for things beyond their control and identification with vulnerable and dependent patients. The pressure to collect data in consultations so that practice targets can be achieved adds to their internal conflict. This may lead to long hours, difficulty in saying 'no' and problems with boundaries.

The second GP has a pragmatic approach and avoids getting embroiled in emotional issues, either their own or those of their patients. This doctor wants patients to let go and not be too needy. Colleagues see them as a sound doctor, but unlikely to be the one who sees the extras, or picks up staff requests to sort out a problem. This GP is perceived to be the one who works hard but always seems to finish on time. They are surprised, maybe angry, when patients do not take their advice. They focus on diagnostics and investigation and good control of long-term conditions. Patients are sometimes reluctant to see them. This doctor risks becoming resentful, irritable and brusque, and dissatisfied with work and the system. Not open to talking about their feelings they risk becoming professionally isolated and lonely. It is easy to see how over time, the first doctor may become emotionally exhausted and the second disillusioned or bored. The wellbeing of both is at risk.

What of the resilient person? Resilience can be defined as a flexible adaptability in the face of challenge, persisting over time. It implies an ability to move forwards in a positive way despite experiencing situations with possible negative outcomes. In our analytic model, this is the person with an adequately nurtured inner self who has the confidence to keep trying, but an appropriate sense of their own efficacy, aware of what they *themselves* can do in the face of challenge and what they can't do. They can manage the anxiety experienced in the face of setbacks without excessive self-blame. Rather than take on excessive responsibility for situations, they may support others, for example patients or team members, to find their own solutions. They can ask others for input or work to change external systems which they find unhelpful.

Though a variety of the characteristics described above can occur in one person, according to circumstances, it is common to see particular attitudes and behaviours repeating. Recognising and understanding our own traits allows us to reflect on our own contribution when we are facing difficult times.

## Why is it so difficult for doctors to ask for help?

There is quite an expectation that doctors will be strong. Patients often need this, team members may expect it, and doctors expect it of themselves. Emotional responses of health professionals to sickness, suffering and death, other than those that offer evidence of strength and capacity, are rarely acknowledged during training and the fact of their existence may be actively denied. In the competitive environment of medicine, it takes courage to be seen as 'sensitive'. The psychoanalytic perspective invites us to consider that the 'strong doctor' projects his or her vulnerable 'weak parts' into the patient in order to preserve an inner sense of potency and strength. Doctors asked to talk about attitudes to their own health or that of colleagues confirm a culture where admitting to illness or stress feels unacceptable. Being the bearer of bad news, invading people's bodies in various ways, listening to distress and being unable to alter the course of nature does require considerable courage. Perhaps it is easier to keep our own vulnerability separate, to deny it, or keep it hidden. We may have concerns about confidentiality, meeting patients in healthcare settings and career damage, especially where mental health or substance abuse problems arise. Then there is strong sense of shame. We should have known better.

## Can resilience be learned, or are we just the way we are?

We each have our own inner world, or mindset, in which we make sense of our experiences and relationships, and that colours our individual responses and decision-making. Knowing something about this inner world, what comes from within ourselves rather than other people, and how this determines our perception and responses to the external world, adds to our resources and enhances resilience. We wrote before about the inner voice, or in analytic language, our superego. Do we recognise a tendency to self-blame when things go wrong, even in circumstances beyond our control, or feel blamed by others and feel rather quickly misunderstood?

We can think about the idea of 'looking after ourselves' as being like a regular consultation between one part of ourselves, the professional, and another part, the patient. This can develop into a space that allows the struggling or suffering part to be heard by the professional part. Questions can be asked, such as 'Do I feel well?', 'Am I taking care of my lifestyle?', 'How are my relationships at work and at home?', 'Am I enjoying my job, or do I recognise a reluctance to see patients?' and 'Do I feel a sense of failure?' It is about knowing ourselves better. Informed by this improved understanding, we are then able to offer ourselves appropriate care and nourishment.

So perhaps resilience can be developed. Part of becoming more resilient is to try to modify the critical voice into something more benign; learning how to feel that being 'good enough' is a realistic aim. In addition, we need to try to be more nurturing of ourselves and accepting of our vulnerabilities and uncertainties. Becoming resilient is also about seeking ways of surrounding ourselves with people who are good for us, at least for some of the time. For some, this may be pursuing a special interest within medicine with like minds, or taking on a management role, or chairing an ethics committee, to create a different work balance. Some people find a 'coaching' approach suits them, which can identify strengths and weaknesses and look for solutions, or new outlets, to create more balance. Self-development can be to improve confidence in parts of work practice that we find difficult, such as time management. There may be a peer group to join, which can bring a new sense of perspective on our own insecurities, often more common than we expect. Some deaneries offer postgraduate courses for cohorts of GPs who study together.

Balint groups offer a place to think about those consultations with patients that leave something uncomfortable lingering in our minds, or where we have a feeling of being stuck or just puzzled. The focus is on the clinician-patient relationship and can be helpful in understanding how the patient's inner world may affect us, and that 'just being there' for the patient may be good enough, if not better, than trying too hard to help. It is not the purpose of Balint groups to scrutinise our inner worlds, or provide therapy, but Michael Balint believed that through a process of self-reflection within the group, a member could undergo a 'small but definite change in personality'. It can help us to see our blind spots. We might recognise how we easily take on a role of rescuer, despite repeated failure of others to succeed, and ask ourselves what this means about our own needs.

What if we recognise a health need? Difficult though it can be to present to another practitioner, the optimal route for care is via a normal patient path, to see a GP. Many doctors are not registered with a GP, or even if they are, tend to self-refer, or self-prescribe. There is some debate about whether there should be more facility for practitioners to self-refer to specific services for doctors, especially where substance abuse or mental health problems are involved. In situations where fitness to practise is at stake, or has already come into play, then it could be argued that this is reasonable, and there are projects taking place on these lines in some parts of the UK. A number of organisations can be contacted in confidence for an initial discussion (see 'Resources' at end of chapter).

What if we want to understand ourselves better, having recognised patterns in our own behaviour, or perhaps some difficult feelings that we would like to try to resolve, but don't want to do this in a professional group? This is where psychotherapy is worth considering, of which there are a number of different modes. There can be a perception that this is just for people with 'much worse problems than mine'. However, we could see it as a private space to get help, to explore ourselves and develop, and a valid way to self-nurture. Considering the complex and emotional work done in primary care, it is remarkable to many other practitioners that GPs do not have supervision, which is mandatory in several professions. So why should we not consider psychotherapy and clinical supervision purely for self-development?

It is worth remembering that many of us work in teams, which for GPs is the practice. Andrew Elder, a retired GP and active Balint leader, has written and spoken about the practice as a secure base for patients, practitioners and staff, and the threat to this brought by recent changes. Increasing external control of how and what primary care does, the division of tasks within teams and reduced face-to-face contact with other professionals in the community, plus a more anonymous referral system into specialist care, risks leaving GPs with feelings of loss of who they are as professionals. Groups of professionals, like families, can have problems of their own but can also be a support for an individual in 'rocky' times. Although there is not space here to go into the detail of group dynamics, or talk about a systems approach, it is worth noting that sometimes a problem that is a function of the group can be felt by, or attributed to a member of the group. In a healthy practice climate, it may be possible to share feelings and observations and work on the real problem within the group, but where this is not possible, self-care for an individual practitioner may be to look for another place to work.

## Summary

The work of clinicians is complex and emotionally demanding. But professionals dedicated to helping others to get better often find it very difficult to recognise their own needs and seek help. GPs who recognise that vulnerability does not only exist within their patients, but within themselves too, can find ways to become more resilient. A variety of formal and informal systems exist to support clinicians.

## Resources

These are a selection of texts and websites, offered as a starting point if you wish to explore further.

### Practical guide to looking after yourself
Firth-Cozens, J. (2010) How to survive in medicine: personally and professionally. Wiley Blackwell, Oxford.
A practical guide written by a leading researcher into doctors' health who followed up a cohort from medical school into their careers.

### Background reading
Henderson, M., Brooks, S.K., del Busso, L. et al. (2012) Shame! Self-stigmatisation as an obstacle to sick doctors returning to work: a qualitative study. BMJ Open 2: e001776. doi:10.1136/bmjopen-2012- 001776.
Howe, A., Smajdor, A. & Stöckl, A. (2012) Towards an understanding of resilience and its relevance to medical training. Medical Education 46: 349–356.

### Websites
### Organisations offering information, support and links
British Medical Association. Doctors' well-being. http://bma.org.uk/practical-support-at-work/doctors-well-being Includes self-assessment of burnout risk and details of a 24-hour counselling and advice service for medical students and doctors (telephone: 08459 200 169).
General Medical Council. Doctors' health concerns: http://www.gmc-uk.org/concerns/doctors_health_concerns.asp On-line guide 'Your health matters'; written for doctors with health concerns, including those referred to the GMC for health-related reasons.
Support 4 Doctors. Homepage: http://www.support4doctors.org A project of the Royal Medical Benevolent Fund. Comprehensive site covering work/life balance, health, careers, education and training. Practical examples and suggestions. Excellent source of links via homepage to other organisations that can help and advise.
British Psychoanalytic Council: http://www.psychoanalytic-council.org
UK Council for Psychotherapy: http://www.psychotherapy.org.uk Sources if you wish to find a psychotherapist.

### Other links
Royal College of General Practitioners: www.rcgp.org.uk/rcgp-near-you.aspx To find your faculty region for courses, events.
Royal College of Nursing. RCN Member Support Services: http://www.rcn.org.uk/support/services.
UK Balint Society: http://balint.co.uk Further information about the society and its activities.

# Appendix 1

| GAD-7 | | | | |
|---|---|---|---|---|
| **Over the <u>last 2 weeks</u>, how often have you been bothered by the following problems?**<br><br>*(Use "✔" to indicate your answer)* | **Not at all** | **Several days** | **More than half the days** | **Nearly every day** |
| 1. Feeling nervous, anxious or on edge | 0 | 1 | 2 | 3 |
| 2. Not being able to stop or control worrying | 0 | 1 | 2 | 3 |
| 3. Worrying too much about different things | 0 | 1 | 2 | 3 |
| 4. Trouble relaxing | 0 | 1 | 2 | 3 |
| 5. Being so restless that it is hard to sit still | 0 | 1 | 2 | 3 |
| 6. Becoming easily annoyed or irritable | 0 | 1 | 2 | 3 |
| 7. Feeling afraid as if something awful might happen | 0 | 1 | 2 | 3 |

*(For office coding: Total Score T____ = ____ + ____ + ____ )*

Interpretation: GAD
Total score >8 suggests Anxiety Disorder or Panic Disorder

GAD7 can be used to monitor progress with cut-offs of:
5 mild anxiety
10 moderate anxiety
15 severe anxiety

*ABC of Anxiety and Depression*, First Edition. Edited by Linda Gask and Carolyn Chew-Graham.
© 2014 John Wiley & Sons, Ltd. Published 2014 by John Wiley & Sons, Ltd.

# Appendix 2

## PATIENT HEALTH QUESTIONNAIRE (PHQ-9)

NAME:_____  DATE:_____

Over the last *2 weeks,* how often have you been bothered by any of the following problems?
*(use "✓" to indicate your answer)*

| | Not at all | Several days | More than half the days | Nearly every day |
|---|---|---|---|---|
| 1. Little interest or pleasure in doing things | 0 | 1 | 2 | 3 |
| 2. Feeling down, depressed, or hopeless | 0 | 1 | 2 | 3 |
| 3. Trouble falling or staying asleep, or sleeping too much | 0 | 1 | 2 | 3 |
| 4. Feeling tired or having little energy | 0 | 1 | 2 | 3 |
| 5. Poor appetite or overeating | 0 | 1 | 2 | 3 |
| 6. Feeling bad about yourself—or that you are a failure or have let yourself or your family down | 0 | 1 | 2 | 3 |
| 7. Trouble concentrating on things, such as reading the newspaper or watching television | 0 | 1 | 2 | 3 |
| 8. Moving or speaking so slowly that other people could have noticed. Or the opposite — being so figety or restless that you have been moving around a lot more than usual | 0 | 1 | 2 | 3 |
| 9. Thoughts that you would be better off dead, or of hurting yourself | 0 | 1 | 2 | 3 |

add columns ____ + ____ + ____

*(Healthcare professional: For interpretation of TOTAL, please refer to accompanying scoring card).*   TOTAL: _____

| | |
|---|---|
| **10.** If you checked off *any problems,* how *difficult* have these problems made it for you to do your work, take care of things at home, or get along with other people? | Not difficult at all _____ <br> Somewhat difficult _____ <br> Very difficult _____ <br> Extremely difficult _____ |

Copyright © 1999 Pfizer Inc. All rights reserved. Reproduced with permission. PRIME-MD© is a trademark of Pfizer Inc.
A2663B 10-04-2005

*ABC of Anxiety and Depression*, First Edition. Edited by Linda Gask and Carolyn Chew-Graham.
© 2014 John Wiley & Sons, Ltd. Published 2014 by John Wiley & Sons, Ltd.

# PHQ-9 Patient Depression Questionnaire

**For initial diagnosis:**

1. Patient completes PHQ-9 Quick Depression Assessment.
2. If there are at least 4 ✓s in the shaded section (including Questions #1 and #2), consider a depressive disorder. Add score to determine severity.

***Consider Major Depressive Disorder***

- if there are at least 5 ✓s in the shaded section (one of which corresponds to Question #1 or #2)

***Consider Other Depressive Disorder***

- if there are 2–4 ✓s in the shaded section (one of which corresponds to Question #1 or #2)

**Note:** Since the questionnaire relies on patient self-report, all responses should be verified by the clinician, and a definitive diagnosis is made on clinical grounds taking into account how well the patient understood the questionnaire, as well as other relevant information from the patient.
Diagnoses of Major Depressive Disorder or Other Depressive Disorder also require impairment of social, occupational, or other important areas of functioning (Question #10) and ruling out normal bereavement, a history of a Manic Episode (Bipolar Disorder), and a physical disorder, medication, or other drug as the biological cause of the depressive symptoms.

**To monitor severity over time for newly diagnosed patients or patients in current treatment for depression:**

1. Patients may complete questionnaires at baseline and at regular intervals (e.g. every 2 weeks) at home and bring them in at their next appointment for scoring or they may complete the questionnaire during each scheduled appointment.
2. Add up ✓s by column. For every ✓: Several days = 1; More than half the days = 2; Nearly every day = 3
3. Add together column scores to get a TOTAL score.
4. Refer to the accompanying **PHQ-9 Scoring Box** to interpret the TOTAL score.
5. Results may be included in patient files to assist you in setting up a treatment goal, determining degree of response, as well as guiding treatment intervention.

**Scoring: add up all checked boxes on PHQ-9**

**For every** ✓ Not at all = 0; Several days = 1;
More than half the days = 2; Nearly every day = 3

**Interpretation of Total Score**

| Total Score | Depression Severity |
|---|---|
| 1–4 | Minimal depression |
| 5–9 | Mild depression |
| 10–14 | Moderate depression |
| 15–19 | Moderately severe depression |
| 20–27 | Severe depression |

PHQ9 Copyright © Pfizer Inc. All rights reserved. Reproduced with permission. PRIME-MD ® is a trademark of Pfizer Inc.

A2662B 10-04-2005

# Appendix 3
# Geriatric Depression Scale GDS30

Patient_____ Examiner_____ Date_____

**Directions to Patient:** Please choose the best answer for how you have felt over the past week.
**Directions to Examiner:** Present questions VERBALLY. Circle answer given by patient. Do not show to patient.

| | | | |
|---|---|---|---|
| 1. | Are you basically satisfied with your life? | yes | **no (1)** |
| 2. | Have you dropped many of your activities and interests? | **yes (1)** | no |
| 3. | Do you feel that your life is empty? | **yes (1)** | no |
| 4. | Do you often get bored? | **yes (1)** | no |
| 5. | Are you hopeful about the future? | yes | **no (1)** |
| 6. | Are you bothered by thoughts you can t get out of your head? | **yes (1)** | no |
| 7. | Are you in good spirits most of the time? | yes | **no (1)** |
| 8. | Are you afraid that something bad is going to happen to you? | **yes (1)** | no |
| 9. | Do you feel happy most of the time? | yes | **no (1)** |
| 10. | Do you often feel helpless? | **yes (1)** | no |
| 11. | Do you often get restless and fidgety? | **yes (1)** | no |
| 12. | Do you prefer to stay at home rather than go out and do things? | **yes (1)** | no |
| 13. | Do you frequently worry about the future? | **yes (1)** | no |
| 14. | Do you feel you have more problems with memory than most? | **yes (1)** | no |
| 15. | Do you think it is wonderful to be alive now? | yes | **no (1)** |
| 16. | Do you feel downhearted and blue? | **yes (1)** | no |
| 17. | Do you feel pretty worthless the way you are now? | **yes (1)** | no |
| 18. | Do you worry a lot about the past? | **yes (1)** | no |
| 19. | Do you find life very exciting? | yes | **no (1)** |
| 20. | Is it hard for you to get started on new projects? | **yes (1)** | no |
| 21. | Do you feel full of energy? | yes | **no (1)** |
| 22. | Do you feel that your situation is hopeless? | **yes (1)** | no |
| 23. | Do you think that most people are better off than you are? | **yes (1)** | no |
| 24. | Do you frequently get upset over little things? | **yes (1)** | no |
| 25. | Do you frequently feel like crying? | **yes (1)** | no |
| 26. | Do you have trouble concentrating? | **yes (1)** | no |
| 27. | Do you enjoy getting up in the morning? | yes | **no (1)** |
| 28. | Do you prefer to avoid social occasions? | **yes (1)** | no |
| 29. | Is it easy for you to make decisions? | yes | **no (1)** |
| 30. | Is your mind as clear as it used to be? | yes | **no (1)** |

**TOTAL: Please sum all bolded answers (worth one point) for a total score. _____**

**Scores: 0 - 9 Normal   10 - 19 Mild Depressive   20 - 30 Severe Depressive**
Source: www.stanford.edu/~ yesavage

*ABC of Anxiety and Depression*, First Edition. Edited by Linda Gask and Carolyn Chew-Graham.
© 2014 John Wiley & Sons, Ltd. Published 2014 by John Wiley & Sons, Ltd.

# Appendix 4
# Abbreviated mental test score (AMTS)

The Abbreviated Mental Test Score (AMTS) was introduced by Hodkinson in 1972 to quickly assess elderly patients for the possibility of dementia. The test has utility across a range of acute and outpatient setting. It takes five minutes to administer and must include all 10 questions. A score of less than 7 or 8 suggests cognitive impairment.

|  | Question | Score 0 or 1 |
|---|---|---|
| 1. | How old are you? | |
| 2. | What is the time (nearest hour)? | |
| 3. | Address for recall at the end of test – this should be repeated by the patient, e.g. 42 West Terrace | |
| 4. | What year is it? | |
| 5. | What is the name of this place? | |
| 6. | Can the patient recognise two relevant persons (e.g. nurse/doctor) | |
| 7. | What was the date of your birth? | |
| 8. | When was the second World War? | |
| 9. | Who is the present Prime Minister? | |
| 10. | Count down from 20 to 1 (no errors, no cues) | |
| **TOTAL CORRECT** | | |

Source: Hodkinson (1972) Evaluation of a mental test score for assessment of mental impairment in the elderly.
*Age and Ageing* 1: 233–8. Reproduced with permission of Oxford University Press.

*ABC of Anxiety and Depression*, First Edition. Edited by Linda Gask and Carolyn Chew-Graham.
© 2014 John Wiley & Sons, Ltd. Published 2014 by John Wiley & Sons, Ltd.

# Appendix 5

## Edinburgh Postnatal Depression Scale[1] (EPDS)

Name: _____     Address: _____

Your Date of Birth: _____     _____

Baby's Date of Birth: _____     Phone: _____

As you are pregnant or have recently had a baby, we would like to know how you are feeling. Please check the answer that comes closest to how you have felt **IN THE PAST 7 DAYS**, not just how you feel today.

Here is an example, already completed.

I have felt happy:
- ☐ Yes, all the time
- ☒ Yes, most of the time    This would mean: "I have felt happy most of the time" during the past week.
- ☐ No, not very often    Please complete the other questions in the same way.
- ☐ No, not at all

In the past 7 days:

1. I have been able to laugh and see the funny side of things
   - ☐ As much as I always could
   - ☐ Not quite so much now
   - ☐ Definitely not so much now
   - ☐ Not at all

2. I have looked forward with enjoyment to things
   - ☐ As much as I ever did
   - ☐ Rather less than I used to
   - ☐ Definitely less than I used to
   - ☐ Hardly at all

*3. I have blamed myself unnecessarily when things went wrong
   - ☐ Yes, most of the time
   - ☐ Yes, some of the time
   - ☐ Not very often
   - ☐ No, never

4. I have been anxious or worried for no good reason
   - ☐ No, not at all
   - ☐ Hardly ever
   - ☐ Yes, sometimes
   - ☐ Yes, very often

*5 I have felt scared or panicky for no very good reason
   - ☐ Yes, quite a lot
   - ☐ Yes, sometimes
   - ☐ No, not much
   - ☐ No, not at all

*6. Things have been getting on top of me
   - ☐ Yes, most of the time I haven't been able to cope at all
   - ☐ Yes, sometimes I haven't been coping as well as usual
   - ☐ No, most of the time I have coped quite well
   - ☐ No, I have been coping as well as ever

*7 I have been so unhappy that I have had difficulty sleeping
   - ☐ Yes, most of the time
   - ☐ Yes, sometimes
   - ☐ Not very often
   - ☐ No, not at all

*8 I have felt sad or miserable
   - ☐ Yes, most of the time
   - ☐ Yes, quite often
   - ☐ Not very often
   - ☐ No, not at all

*9 I have been so unhappy that I have been crying
   - ☐ Yes, most of the time
   - ☐ Yes, quite often
   - ☐ Only occasionally
   - ☐ No, never

*10 The thought of harming myself has occurred to me
   - ☐ Yes, quite often
   - ☐ Sometimes
   - ☐ Hardly ever
   - ☐ Never

Administered/Reviewed by _____     Date _____

[1]Source: Cox, J.L., Holden, J.M., and Sagovsky, R. 1987. Detection of postnatal depression: Development of the 10-item Edinburgh Postnatal Depression Scale. *British Journal of Psychiatry* 150:782-786 .

[2]Source: K. L. Wisner, B. L. Parry, C. M. Piontek, Postpartum Depression N Engl J Med vol. 347, No 3, July 18, 2002, 194-199

Users may reproduce the scale without further permission providing they respect copyright by quoting the names of the authors, the title and the source of the paper in all reproduced copies.

*ABC of Anxiety and Depression*, First Edition. Edited by Linda Gask and Carolyn Chew-Graham.
© 2014 John Wiley & Sons, Ltd. Published 2014 by John Wiley & Sons, Ltd.

# Edinburgh Postnatal Depression Scale[1] (EPDS)

Postpartum depression is the most common complication of childbearing.[2] The 10-question Edinburgh Postnatal Depression Scale (EPDS) is a valuable and efficient way of identifying patients at risk for "perinatal" depression. The EPDS is easy to administer and has proven to be an effective screening tool.

Mothers who score above 13 are likely to be suffering from a depressive illness of varying severity. The EPDS score should not override clinical judgment. A careful clinical assessment should be carried out to confirm the diagnosis. The scale indicates how the mother has felt *during the previous week*. In doubtful cases it may be useful to repeat the tool after 2 weeks. The scale will not detect mothers with anxiety neuroses, phobias or personality disorders.

Women with postpartum depression need not feel alone. They may find useful information on the web sites of the National Women's Health Information Center <www.4women.gov> and from groups such as Postpartum Support International <www.chss.iup.edu/postpartum> and Depression after Delivery <www.depressionafterdelivery.com>.

---

## SCORING

**QUESTIONS 1, 2, & 4 (without an *)**
Are scored 0, 1, 2 or 3 with top box scored as 0 and the bottom box scored as 3.

**QUESTIONS 3, 5-10 (marked with an *)**
Are reverse scored, with the top box scored as a 3 and the bottom box scored as 0.

      Maximum score:      30
      Possible Depression:  10 or greater
      Always look at item 10 (suicidal thoughts)

Users may reproduce the scale without further permission, providing they respect copyright by quoting the names of the authors, the title, and the source of the paper in all reproduced copies.

---

## Instructions for using the Edinburgh Postnatal Depression Scale:

1. The mother is asked to check the response that comes closest to how she has been feeling in the previous 7 days.

2. All the items must be completed.

3. Care should be taken to avoid the possibility of the mother discussing her answers with others. (Answers come from the mother or pregnant woman.)

4. The mother should complete the scale herself, unless she has limited English or has difficulty with reading.

---

[1]Source: Cox, J.L., Holden, J.M., and Sagovsky, R. 1987. Detection of postnatal depression: Development of the 10-item Edinburgh Postnatal Depression Scale. *British Journal of Psychiatry* 150:782-786.

[2]Source: K. L. Wisner, B. L. Parry, C. M. Piontek, Postpartum Depression N Engl J Med vol. 347, No 3, July 18, 2002, 194-199

# Appendix 6

## Hospital Anxiety and Depression Scale

This questionnaire helps your physician to know how you are feeling. Read every sentence. Place an "X" on the answer that best describes how you have been feeling during the LAST WEEK. You do not have to think too much to answer. In this questionnaire, spontaneous answers are more important

| A | I feel tense or 'wound up': | |
|---|---|---|
| | Most of the time | 3 |
| | A lot of the time | 2 |
| | From time to time (acc.) | 1 |
| | Not at all | 0 |

| D | I still enjoy the things I used to enjoy: | |
|---|---|---|
| | Definitely as much | 0 |
| | Not quite as much | 1 |
| | Only a little | 2 |
| | Hardly at all | 3 |

| A | I get a sort of frightened feeling as if something awful is about to happen: | |
|---|---|---|
| | Very definitely and quite badly | 3 |
| | yes, but not too badly | 2 |
| | A little, but it doesn't worry me | 1 |
| | Not at all | 0 |

| D | I can laugh and see the funny side of things: | |
|---|---|---|
| | As much as I always could | 0 |
| | Not quite so much now | 1 |
| | Definitely not so much now | 2 |
| | Not at all | 3 |

| A | Worrying thoughts go through my mind: | |
|---|---|---|
| | A great deal of the time | 3 |
| | A lot of the time | 2 |
| | From time to time, but not often | 1 |
| | Only occasionally | 0 |

| D | I feel cheerful: | |
|---|---|---|
| | Not at all | 3 |
| | Not often | 2 |
| | Sometimes | 1 |
| | Most of the time | 0 |

| A | I can sit at ease and feet relaxed: | |
|---|---|---|
| | Definitely | 0 |
| | Usually | 1 |
| | Not often | 2 |
| | Not at all | 3 |

| D | I feel as if I am slowed down: | |
|---|---|---|
| | Nearly all the time | 3 |
| | Very often | 2 |
| | Sometimes | 1 |
| | Not at all | 0 |

| A | I get a sort of frightened feeling like "butterflies" in the stomach: | |
|---|---|---|
| | Not at all | 0 |
| | Occasionally | 1 |
| | Quite often | 2 |
| | Very often | 3 |

| D | I have lost interest in my appearance: | |
|---|---|---|
| | Definitely | 3 |
| | I don't take as much care as I should | 2 |
| | I may not take quite as much care | 1 |
| | I take just as much care | 0 |

| A | I feel restless as I have to be on the move: | |
|---|---|---|
| | Very much indeed | 3 |
| | Quite a lot | 2 |
| | Not very much | 1 |
| | Not at all | 0 |

| D | I look forward with enjoyment to things: | |
|---|---|---|
| | As much as I ever did | 0 |
| | Rather less than I used to | 1 |
| | Definitely less than I used to | 2 |
| | Hardly at all | 3 |

| A | I get sudden feelings of panic: | |
|---|---|---|
| | Very often indeed | 3 |
| | Quite often | 2 |
| | Not very often | 1 |
| | Not at all | 0 |

| D | I can enjoy a good book or radio/TV program: | |
|---|---|---|
| | Often | 0 |
| | Sometimes | 1 |
| | Not often | 2 |
| | Very seldom | 3 |

## Scoring

HADS has 14 items, seven of which are aimed at evaluating anxiety, marked by the letter A (HADS-A), and seven for depression. marked by the letter D (HADS-D). Each item receives a score that ranges from 0–3, achieving a maximal scorc of 21 points for each scale.
- HADS-A (Anxiety): 0–8 without anxiety, ≥9 with anxiety
- HADS-D (Depression ): 0–8 without depression, ≥9 with depression

Source: Zigmond & Snalth, 1983. Acta Psychiatrica Scandinavica 67: 361–370. Reproduced with permission from Wiley.

*ABC of Anxiety and Depression*, First Edition. Edited by Linda Gask and Carolyn Chew-Graham.
© 2014 John Wiley & Sons, Ltd. Published 2014 by John Wiley & Sons, Ltd.

# Appendix 7

**MONTREAL COGNITIVE ASSESSMENT (MOCA)**
Version 7.1 Original Version

NAME :
Education :          Date of birth :
Sex :          DATE :

| VISUOSPATIAL / EXECUTIVE | | POINTS |
|---|---|---|

Copy cube

Draw CLOCK (Ten past eleven) ( 3 points )

(E) End  (A)
(5)
(1) Begin  (B)  (2)
(D)  (4)  (3)
(C)

[ ]          [ ]          [ ]  [ ]  [ ]    __/5
Contour  Numbers  Hands

**NAMING**

[ ]          [ ]          [ ]    __/3

| MEMORY | Read list of words, subject must repeat them. Do 2 trials, even if 1st trial is successful. Do a recall after 5 minutes. | | FACE | VELVET | CHURCH | DAISY | RED | No points |
|---|---|---|---|---|---|---|---|---|
| | | 1st trial | | | | | | |
| | | 2nd trial | | | | | | |

| ATTENTION | Read list of digits (1 digit/ sec.). | Subject has to repeat them in the forward order | [ ] 2 1 8 5 4 | __/2 |
|---|---|---|---|---|
| | | Subject has to repeat them in the backward order | [ ] 7 4 2 | |

Read list of letters. The subject must tap with his hand at each letter A. No points if ≥ 2 errors
[ ]  F B A C M N A A J K L B A F A K D E A A A J A M O F A A B          __/1

Serial 7 subtraction starting at 100    [ ] 93    [ ] 86    [ ] 79    [ ] 72    [ ] 65    __/3
4 or 5 correct subtractions: **3 pts**, 2 or 3 correct: **2 pts**, 1 correct: **1 pt**, 0 correct: **0 pt**

| LANGUAGE | Repeat : I only know that John is the one to help today. [ ] The cat always hid under the couch when dogs were in the room. [ ] | __/2 |
|---|---|---|

Fluency / Name maximum number of words in one minute that begin with the letter F    [ ] _____ (N ≥ 11 words)    __/1

**ABSTRACTION**    Similarity between e.g. banana - orange = fruit    [ ] train – bicycle    [ ] watch - ruler    __/2

| DELAYED RECALL | Has to recall words **WITH NO CUE** | FACE [ ] | VELVET [ ] | CHURCH [ ] | DAISY [ ] | RED [ ] | Points for UNCUED recall only | __/5 |
|---|---|---|---|---|---|---|---|---|
| **Optional** | Category cue | | | | | | | |
| | Multiple choice cue | | | | | | | |

**ORIENTATION**    [ ] Date    [ ] Month    [ ] Year    [ ] Day    [ ] Place    [ ] City    __/6

© Z.Nasreddine MD          www.mocatest.org          Normal ≥26 / 30    TOTAL    __/30
Administered by: _____          Add 1 point if ≤ 12 yr edu

Source: http://www.mocatest.org/. Reproduced with permission of Dr Z. Nasreddine.

*ABC of Anxiety and Depression*, First Edition. Edited by Linda Gask and Carolyn Chew-Graham.
© 2014 John Wiley & Sons, Ltd. Published 2014 by John Wiley & Sons, Ltd.

# Appendix 8

## ADDENBROOKE'S COGNITIVE EXAMINATION – ACE-R

### *Administration and Scoring Guide - 2006*

The ACE-R[1] is a brief cognitive test that assesses five cognitive domains, namely attention/orientation, memory, verbal fluency, language and visuospatial abilities. Total score is 100, higher scores indicates better cognitive functioning.

Administration of the ACE-R takes, on average, 15 minutes.

These instructions have been designed in order to make the questions and their scoring clear for the tester. Please read them carefully before giving the test.

If possible, leave the scoring until the end of the session, since the participant will not be able to check whether the tester is ticking for correct answers or crossing for wrong ones. This might avoid anxiety, which can disturb the participant's performance on the test.

### ORIENTATION – score 0 to 10

Ask the participant for the day, date, month, year and season. Score one point for each correct answer.

Ask the participant for the name of the hospital (or building), the floor (or room), the town, county and country. Score one point for each correct answer.

Record responses. Allow mistakes for the date (+ or – 2 days). If assessing a participant at home, ask for the name of the place i.e. name of the house e.g. "The Gables", and for the floor you might ask for the name of the room (kitchen, living room, etc). If at a single storey health setting, ask about a local landmark. When the season is changing, e.g. at the end of August, and the participant says "autumn", ask them "could it be another season?". If answer is "summer", give one point, since the two seasons are in transition. Do not give one point if the answer is "winter" or "spring".

*Seasons*: spring - March, April, May; summer - June, July, August; autumn - September, October, November; winter - December, January, February.

### REGISTRATION – score 0 to 3

Ask the participant to repeat and remember the words lemon, key, and ball. Speak slowly. Repeat them if necessary (maximum 3 times). Tell the participant that you will ask for this information later. Record the number of trials. Score the first attempt only.

### ATTENTION & CONCENTRATION – score 0 to 5

*Calculation*: Ask the participant to subtract 7 from 100, record the answer, then ask them to subtract 7 from that, record the answer. Do this 5 times. If the participant makes a mistake, carry on and check subsequent answers for scoring. Record responses (Example: 92, 85, 79, 72, 65, score 3).

*Spelling*: give this test if the participant makes a mistake on the calculation task. Start by asking the participant to spell "world". Then ask them to spell it backwards. Record responses.

Scoring for the spelling task:
- Score 1 point for each correct letter spelt. Correct sequence = D L R O W = 5 points
- Count one error for each omission, letter transposition (switching adjacent letters), insertion (inserting a new letter), or misplacement (moving W, O, R, L, D by more than one space).

**Examples (score in parentheses):**

Copyright 2000, John Hodges

Source: http://www.neura.edu.au/. Reproduced with permission of Professor John Hodges.

*ABC of Anxiety and Depression*, First Edition. Edited by Linda Gask and Carolyn Chew-Graham.
© 2014 John Wiley & Sons, Ltd. Published 2014 by John Wiley & Sons, Ltd.

|  | omission | transposition | insertion | misplacement |
|---|---|---|---|---|
| omission | DLOW (4) |  |  |  |
| transposition | D*OL*W (3) | DL*OR*W (4) |  |  |
|  | omission | transposition | insertion | misplacement |
| insertion | DL*T*OW (3) | DLR*WWO* (3) | DL*RR*OW(4) |  |
| misplacement | LOW*D* (3) | LR*WOD* (3) | LR*WOWD* (3) | LROW*D* (4) |

A response such as 'LRWWOD' has 3 errors (L and R are correct, for a score of 2). It includes transposition of the W and O, insertion of an extra W, and misplacement of the D. If the patient adds 1 or more of the same letter at the end of the word, count as one error (e.g. ' LDROWWW, would be 2 errors, 1 transposition and 1 addition).

Score one point for each correct calculation or letter spelt. Score only the better performed one.

## R E C A L L – score 0 to 3

Ask the participant to recall the words that you asked them to repeat and remember.
Record responses. Score one point for each correct item.

## Anterograde Memory – score 0 to 7

Instruct the participant: "I'm going to read you a name and address that I'd like you to repeat after me. We'll be doing that 3 times, so you have a chance to learn it. I'll be asking you about it later". If the participant starts repeating along with you, ask them to wait until you give it in full.
Record responses for each trial. However, only the third score contributes to the ACE-R score (0-7points).

## Retrograde Memory – score 0 to 4

Ask the participant for the name of the current Prime Minister, the woman who was Prime Minister, the president of the US and the president of the US who was assassinated in the sixties.
Score one point each. Allow answers like Blair, Thatcher; Bush; Kennedy. Do not accept answers like Maggie, ask for surname as well.

## V E R B A L   F L U E N C Y – score 0 to 14

### Letters – score 0 to 7

Instruct the participant: "I'm going to give you a letter of the alphabet and I'd like you to generate as many words as you can beginning with that letter, but not the names of people or places. Are you ready? You've got a minute and the letter is P".
Participant might repeat or perseverate words, e.g. pay, paid, pays. Record and count them for the overall total number of responses but do not consider them for the final score. In the same way, intrusions such as words beginning with other letters are recorded but not scored. Proper names (Peter, Peterborough) do not count. For plurals e.g. pot, pots, total = 2, correct = 1. Use the table provided on the ACE-R sheet to obtain the final score for this test.

### Animals – score 0 to 7

Instruct the participant: "Now can you name as many animals as possible, beginning with any letter?"
Participant might repeat words. Record and count them for the overall total number of responses, but they should not be considered for the final score. The participant may misunderstand and perseverate by naming animals beginning with "p". Repeat instructions during the 60 seconds if necessary.
If subject says e.g. "fish", and later says "salmon" and "trout", count and record as 3 for "total" but do not accept "fish" as correct (count only 2 out of the 3, e.g. "salmon" and "trout"). However, if only the category is given, e.g. fish, with no specific exemplars, then count fish as 1 for total and final correct responses. The same applies to mammals, reptiles, birds, breeds of dog, insects, etc.

Copyright 2000, John Hodges

**L A N G U A G E** - Comprehension (Close your eyes) – score 0 or 1

Instruct the participant: "Read this sentence and do as it says". If the participant reads sentence aloud but does not follow the instructions, score 0.

**L A N G U A G E** - Comprehension (3-stage command) - score 0 to 3

Instruct the participant: "Take this paper in your right hand, fold it in half, and put it on the floor". Do not allow participant to take the paper before you have finished giving the complete instruction.
Score one point for each correct command, e.g. if participant takes the paper and puts it on the floor without folding, score 2; if participant takes the paper in their right hand, and folds it several times and leaves on the table, score 1.

**L A N G U A G E** - Writing – score 0 or 1

Instruct the participant to write a sentence.
The sentence should contain a subject and a verb, and it should have a meaning.
Do not accept "Happy Birthday" or "Nice day" as a sentence. If participant has difficulty thinking of something to write, prompt gently with "What's the weather like today?"

**L A N G U A G E** - Repetition – score 0 to 2

Ask the participant to repeat the words after you. Say one word at a time. Circle the words that were repeated incorrectly. Consider first attempt only for scoring. Record responses. Score 2 if all words are correct; 1 if 3 are correct; 0 if 2 or less are correct.

**L A N G U A G E** - Repetition – score 0 to 2

Ask the participant to repeat each sentence. Do not accept partially correct repetitions, e.g. "no ifs and buts", "above below" as correct for scoring. Score one point for each sentence.

**L A N G U A G E** - Naming – score 0 to 2

**Naming (watch and pencil)**
Ask the participant to name each picture. Correct answers: pencil; wristwatch or watch.

**L A N G U A G E** - Naming – score 0 to 10

**Naming (5 animals and 5 objects)**
Ask the participant to name each picture. Correct answers: penguin; anchor; camel or dromedary; barrel or tub; crown; crocodile or alligator; harp; rhinoceros or rhino; kangaroo or wallaby; piano accordion, accordion or squeeze box.
Score one point each.

**L A N G U A G E** - Comprehension – score 0 to 4

**Comprehension**
Ask the participant to point to the pictures according to the statement read.
Score one point each. Allow self-corrections.

Copyright 2000, John Hodges

## LANGUAGE - Reading – score 0 or 1

Ask the participant to read the words aloud. Score one point only if all five words are correctly read. Record the mistakes using the phonetic alphabet if possible.

## VISUOSPATIAL ABILITIES - Overlapping pentagons – score 0 or 1

The pentagons should clearly show 5 sides and the intersection.

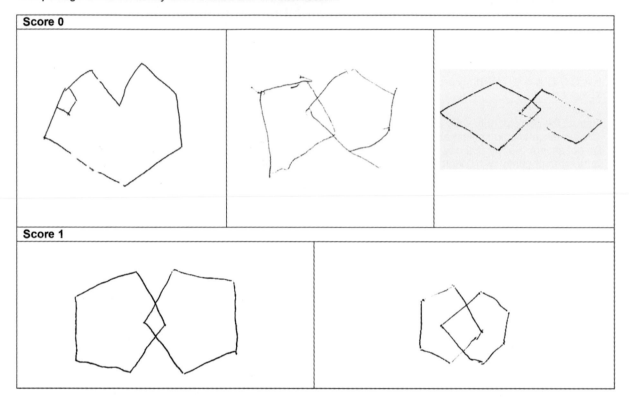

## VISUOSPATIAL ABILITIES - Wire Cube – score 0 to 2

Cube should have 12 lines = score 2, even if the proportions are not perfect. A score of 1 is given if cube has fewer than 12 lines, but general cube shape is maintained. See examples below.

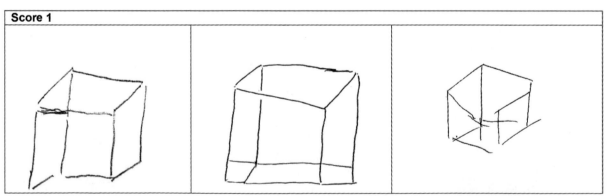

Copyright 2000, John Hodges

**Score 2**

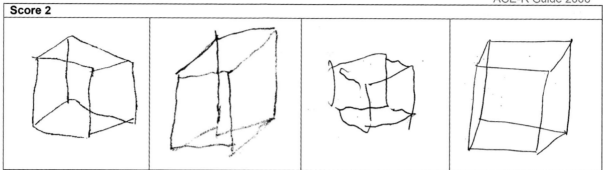

## VISUOSPATIAL ABILITIES - Clock – score 0 to 5

Ask the participant to draw a clock face with the numbers on it. When he/she has finished, ask them to put the hands at "ten past five".

| | |
|---|---|
| **Circle** | 1 point maximum if it is a reasonable circle |
| **Numbers** | 2 points if all included and well distributed<br>1 point if all included but poorly distributed |
| **Hands** | 2 points if both hands are well drawn, different lengths and placed on correct numbers (you might ask which one is the small and big one)<br>1point if both placed on the correct numbers but wrong lengths OR<br>1 point if one hand is placed on the correct number and drawn with correct length OR<br>1 point if only one hand is drawn and placed at the correct number i.e. 5 for 'ten past five' |

**Score 2**

Circle (1), one hand placed correctly (1)

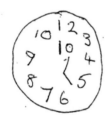

Circle (1); all the numbers but not placed inside the circle (1)

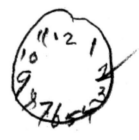

**Score 3**

Circle (1); all the numbers but not proportionally distributed (1), one hand placed correctly (1)

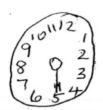

Circle (1), all the numbers but not placed inside the circle (1), one hand place correctly (1).

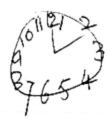

Circle (1), note that numbers are not inside the circle and there are 2 number 10s (0), hands placed correctly

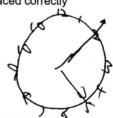

Copyright 2000, John Hodges

ACE-R Guide 2006

| Score 4 | | |
|---|---|---|
| Circle(1); numbers proportionally distributed (2); one hand placed correctly (1) | Circle (1); all the numbers but not proportionally distributed (1); both hands placed correctely (2) | Circle (1); numbers proportionally distributed (2), one hand placed correctly (1) |
| 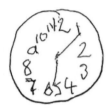 | 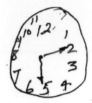 | 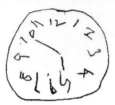 |

| Score 5 |
|---|
| Circle (1); numbers proportionally distributed on both halves of the clock face (2); hands placed correctly (2) |
| 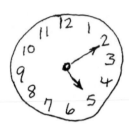 |

## PERCEPTUAL ABILITIES – score 0 to 4

**Counting dots**
Participant is *not* allowed to point to the picture. Score one point for each correct answer.
Correct answers, from top left clockwise: 8, 10, 9 and 7.

## PERCEPTUAL ABILITIES – score 0 to 4

**Identifying letters**
Participant is allowed to point to the picture. Score one point for each correct answer.
Correct answers, from top left clockwise: K, M, T and A

## RECALL – score 0 to 7

**Recall**
Say to the participant: "Now tell me what you remember of that name and address we were repeating at the beginning". Tick and score one point for each item recalled, using the score guide provided in the test.

**Harry Barnes
73 Orchard Close
Kingsbridge
Devon**

**Example 1a**

| Harry Bond | 1 + 0 | |
|---|---|---|
| 78 Orchard Close | 0 + 1 + 1 | |
| Kingsbury | 0 | |
| …. | 0 | **Score 3/7** |

Copyright 2000, John Hodges

ACE-R Guide 2006

**Example 2a**

| Harry Barnes | 1 + 1 | |
|---|---|---|
| 73 Kingsbridge Close | 1 + 0 + 1 | |
| .... | 0 | |
| Devon | 1 | **Score 5/7** |

**Example 3a**

| Harry Bond | 1 + 0 | |
|---|---|---|
| 33 Kingsbury Way | 0 + 0 + 0 | |
| Kingsbridge Close | 0 + 0 | |
| Cambridge | 0 | |
| Devon | 1 | **Score 2/7** |

## RECOGNITION – score 0 to 5

**Recognition – only to be given if participant fails to recall one or more items in the recall task.**
This task should be given to allow the participant a chance to recognise items that he or she could not recall. If the participant recalls the name and address correctly, this test is not needed and the participant scores 5. However, many participants will recall only parts. Start by ticking the correctly remembered items on the shadowed column (right hand side) and then tell them "Let me give you some hints. Was the number (or whatever was forgotten or mistaken) x, y or z?" and so on. Every recognised item scores one point. Maximum score is 5. Adding recalled items to those recognised gives the final score for this part of the test.

**Example 1b (based on example 1a)**

| Tester ticks "Orchard Close" on the right hand side shadowed column because participant had recalled that item. The tester should then ask:<br><br>- Was it Jerry Barnes, <u>Harry Barnes</u> or Harry Bradford?<br>- Was it 37, <u>73</u> or 76?<br>- Was it Oakhampton, <u>Kingsbridge</u> or Dartington?<br>- Was it <u>Devon</u>, Dorset or Somerset? | Participant's answers:<br><br>Harry Barnes<br>76<br>Kingsbridge<br>Dorset | <br><br>1<br>0<br>1<br>0<br>+ 1 (Orchard Close)<br><br>**Score 3/5** |
|---|---|---|

**Example 2b (based on example 2a)**

| Tester ticks "Harry Barnes", "73" and "Devon" on the right hand side shadowed column because participant had recalled those items. The tester should then ask:<br><br>- Was it Orchard Place, Oak Close or <u>Orchard Close</u>?<br>- Was it Oakhampton, <u>Kingsbridge</u> or Dartington? | Participant's answers:<br><br>Orchard Close<br><br>Kingsbridge | <br><br>1<br><br>1<br><br>+ 3 (Harry Barnes, 73, Devon)<br><br>**Score 5/5** |
|---|---|---|

**Example 3b (based on example 3a)**

| Tester ticks "Devon", on the right hand side shadowed column because participant had recalled that item. The tester should then ask:<br><br>- Was it Jerry Barnes, <u>Harry Barnes</u> or Harry Bradford?<br>- Was it 37, <u>73</u> or 76?<br>- Was it <u>Orchard Place</u>, Oak Close or Orchard Close?<br>- Was it Oakhampton, <u>Kingsbridge</u> or Dartington? | Participant's answers:<br><br>Jerry Barnes<br><br>37<br>Orchard Place<br><br>Oakhampton | <br><br>0<br><br>0<br>0<br><br>0<br>+1 (Devon)<br>**Score 1/5** |
|---|---|---|

Copyright 2000, John Hodges

## M M S E – score 0 to 30

The MMSE score can be obtained by adding up the scores in the shaded boxes to the right hand side of each test.

## NORMATIVE DATA

A total of 241 subjects participated[1], consisting of three groups: a dementia group (n=142), a mild cognitive impairment group (n=36) and a control group (63).

Table 1: Lower limit of normal (cut-off scores) for total ACE-R and sub-scores according to age (50-59, 60-69, 70-75), showing control mean minus two standard deviations.

| Age range | Education (years) | Total ACE-R score | Attention/ Orientation | Memory | Fluency | Language | Visuospatial |
|-----------|------------------|-------------------|------------------------|--------|---------|----------|--------------|
| **50-59** | 12.7 | 86 | 17 | 18 | 9 | 24 | 15 |
| **60-69** | 12.9 | 85 | 17 | 19 | 8 | 21 | 14 |
| **70-75** | 12.1 | 84 | 16 | 17 | 9 | 22 | 14 |

Table 2: Sensitivity, Specificity and Positive Predictive Values (PPV) at different prevalence rates of two cut-off total ACE-R scores. Values in parenthesis represent the respective Negative Predictive Values

|  | **Dementia** |  | PPV at different prevalence rates |  |  |  |
|--|-------------|--|-----------------------------------|--|--|--|
| **ACE-R cut-off** | **Sensitivity** | **Specificity** | **5%** | **10%** | **20%** | **40%** |
| **88** | 0.94 | 0.89 | 0.31 (1.0) | 0.48 | 0.68 | 0.85 (1.0) |
| **82** | 0.84 | 1.00 | 1.0 (0.96) | 1.0 | 1.0 | 1.0 (0.90) |

## Reference

1. Mioshi E, Dawson K, Mitchell J, Arnold R, Hodges JR (2006) The Addenbrooke's Cognitive Examination Revised (ACE-R): a brief cognitive test battery for dementia screening, International Journal of Geriatric Psychiatry (in press).

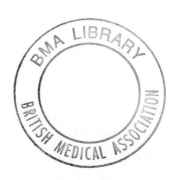

BMA LIBRARY BRITISH MEDICAL ASSOCIATION

Copyright 2000, John Hodges

# Index

Note: Page numbers in *italics* refer to Figures.

*ABC of Anxiety and Depression*, First Edition. Edited by Linda Gask and Carolyn Chew-Graham.
© 2014 John Wiley & Sons, Ltd. Published 2014 by John Wiley & Sons, Ltd.